MAI[illegible] FIRST YEAR OF RETIREMENT UNFORGETTABLE

The Best Unique and Fun Activities to Make the Most of Your Newfound Freedom

HARRY THOMPSON

DJTS PUBLISHING

Contents

INTRODUCTION: WELCOME TO RETIREMENT

Congratulations on reaching retirement! This is the beginning of a new and exciting chapter in your life. You've worked hard for many years, and now it's time to relax and enjoy the fruits of your labor.

Retirement can be a daunting prospect, but it doesn't have to be. In fact, retirement can be one of the most fulfilling and enjoyable periods of your life. It's a time to pursue your passions, spend time with loved ones, travel, and try new things.

In this book, we'll explore fun and unique activities that will make your first year of retirement unforgettable. From learning a new language to starting a garden, there's something for everyone in these pages.

But before we dive into all the exciting activities that await you in retirement, let's take a moment to reflect on what this milestone means. Retirement isn't just about leaving work behind; it's about embarking on a new phase of life filled with endless possibilities.

So, take a deep breath and savor this moment. You've earned it. And get ready for an adventure unlike any other - one that will leave you feeling fulfilled, happy, and grateful every day.

Let's get started!

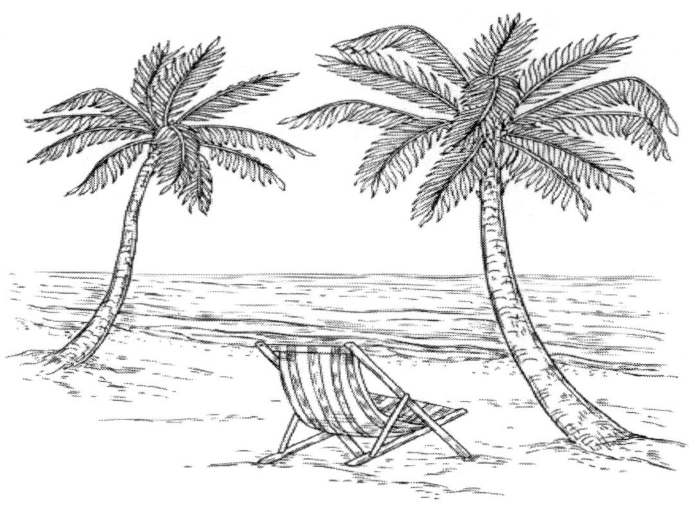

UNFORGETTABLE ADVENTURES

Embark on exciting and memorable adventures during your first year of retirement. This chapter will guide you through unique and fun activities that will help you make the most of your newfound freedom. From thrilling outdoor experiences to cultural explorations, this chapter has something for everyone looking to add some excitement to their retirement years. Get ready to create unforgettable memories with these adventurous activities.

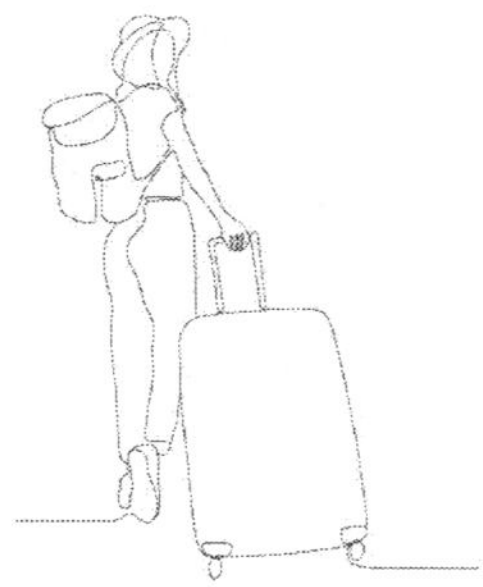

Traveling the World

Are you ready to take off and explore the world in your retirement? We'll take a look at some of the most exciting and fulfilling ways to experience new cultures, cuisines, and landscapes. Whether you're looking for adventure or relaxation, there's something for everyone on our list of travel activities. So pack your bags and get ready to embark on an unforgettable journey!

- **Volunteer Tourism -** Make a difference while seeing the world by participating in volunteer tourism. Help build homes, teach children, or work on conservation projects in foreign countries. Not only will you have a meaningful experience, but you'll also gain insight into different cultures and make new friends along the way.

- **Culinary Tours -** Food is one of the best ways to experience a culture, so why not take a culinary tour of a foreign country? Learn how to cook traditional dishes, sample local delicacies, and even visit markets to learn about ingredients used in regional cuisine.

- **House-Sitting -** Want to live like a local instead of staying at a hotel? Consider house-sitting for someone while they're away on vacation. You'll get free accommodation in exchange for taking care of their home and pets. This is a great option if you want an extended stay in one location.

- **Train Journeys -** Take the scenic route by embarking on a train journey through beautiful landscapes. From the Orient Express in Europe to the Trans-Siberian Railway in Russia, there are plenty of options for train travel that will take you through stunning scenery and allow you to see parts of the world that may be difficult to access otherwise.

- **Cultural Festivals -** Experience a country's unique traditions and customs by attending cultural festivals around the world. From Dia de los Muertos in Mexico to Holi Festival in India, there's no shortage of celebrations that offer insight into different cultures.

- **Road Trips -** Take a classic American road trip or venture out on a scenic drive in another country. Rent an RV or car and hit the open road to discover hidden gems and breathtaking views along the way.

- **Homestays -** Similar to house-sitting, homestays allow you to immerse yourself in local culture by staying with a host family.

You'll get a taste of daily life and have the opportunity to learn about customs and traditions firsthand.

- **Wellness Retreats -** Combine travel with self-care by attending a wellness retreat abroad. From yoga retreats in Bali to meditation retreats in India, there are plenty of options for rejuvenating your mind, body, and soul while exploring new destinations.
- **Eco-Tourism -** If you're passionate about sustainability and conservation, consider eco-tourism as your next travel adventure. Visit national parks, wildlife reserves, or participate in conservation projects that help protect endangered species around the world.
- **Cruise Ship Adventures -** Take advantage of all-inclusive amenities while exploring multiple destinations on a cruise ship adventure. Choose from river cruises in Europe or ocean cruises through Asia or South America for an unforgettable experience.
- **Trekking -** If you're looking for an adventure that combines hiking with stunning scenery, trekking might be for you. From the Inca Trail in Peru to the Himalayas in Nepal, there are plenty of options for trekking destinations around the world that offer breathtaking views and a sense of accomplishment.
- **Language Immersion Programs -** If you've always wanted to learn a new language or improve your fluency in one, consider attending a language immersion program abroad. You'll have the opportunity to practice speaking with native speakers and immerse yourself in local culture while learning.

- **Agritourism -** For those interested in agriculture and farming, agritourism offers opportunities to visit working farms and vineyards around the world. Learn about local food production methods, try fresh produce straight from the source, and even participate in farm activities like grape picking or cheese making.

- **Adventure Sports -** From skiing in the Swiss Alps to surfing in Costa Rica, adventure sports offer exciting ways to explore new destinations while getting your adrenaline pumping. Try something new like bungee jumping or paragliding for a truly unforgettable experience.

- **Cultural Tours -** To gain deeper insights into different cultures around the world, consider taking cultural tours that focus on specific aspects of a country's history and traditions. Examples include visiting ancient temples in Asia or exploring art museums throughout Europe.

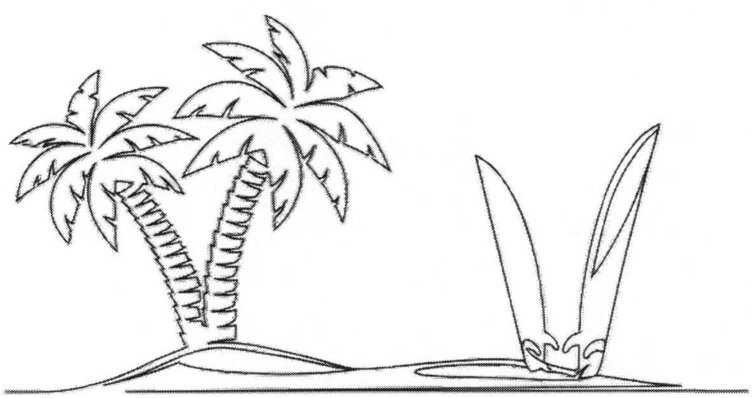

Embracing the Great Outdoors

There's something special about being surrounded by nature, especially as you begin this new chapter in your life. In this chapter, we'll explore different ways to connect with the great outdoors and make unforgettable memories. From scenic hikes to wildlife encounters, get ready to embrace the beauty of nature and all it has to offer.

- **Forest Bathing - Have you heard of forest bathing?** It's a Japanese practice that involves immersing yourself in nature by taking long walks in the woods. Not only is it a great way to get exercise, but studies have shown that spending time in nature can also reduce stress levels and improve mental clarity. So why not try it out for yourself? Find a local park or hiking trail, put on your walking shoes, and take in all the sights, sounds, and smells of nature.

- **Birdwatching -** Birdwatching is another great way to get outside and enjoy nature. It's a peaceful activity that allows you to observe birds in their natural habitats while also getting some fresh air and exercise. You don't need any special equipment to start birdwatching – just grab a pair of binoculars and head outside.

- **Kayaking -** Kayaking is an excellent way to explore bodies of water such as rivers, lakes or oceans whilst enjoying the beauty surrounding them from up close at your own pace. Whether you're paddling through calm waters or navigating rapids - kayaking provides both an adrenaline rush and peaceful tranquility.

- **Stargazing -** Stargazing is an ideal way to spend evenings outdoors with family or friends during summers especially when there are meteor showers going on or constellations are visible clearly from where you live! Take blankets, snacks along with telescopes if possible - sit back & relax while exploring the universe from your backyard!

- **Rock Climbing -** Rock climbing is a thrilling way to get outside and challenge yourself physically, while also appreciating the beauty of natural rock formations. There are many options for indoor or outdoor climbing, as well as varying levels of difficulty for climbers of all abilities. If you're new to rock climbing, consider taking a class or hiring a guide to ensure safety and proper technique.

- **Wildlife Photography -** If you have an interest in photography, combining it with nature can result in stunning images that will last forever! Wildlife photography is an excellent way to capture the beauty of animals in their natural habitats while also getting some exercise outdoors. You don't need any fancy equipment to start wildlife photography – just grab your camera or smartphone and head outside on a hike or nature walk.

- **Beachcombing -** Beachcombing involves exploring the shorelines of beaches for interesting shells, rocks, driftwood or even sea glass! It's a great way to get some fresh air and exercise while also discovering unique treasures from the beach. Make sure to bring along a bag or bucket to collect your finds!

- **Outdoor Yoga -** Outdoor yoga allows you to connect with nature whilst practicing mindfulness & meditation in serene environments such as parks or gardens. The fresh air & calming sounds of nature make it an ideal setting for rejuvenating body & soul. Many communities offer free outdoor yoga classes so check local listings online!

- **Horseback Riding -** Horseback riding is an enjoyable activity that provides both physical exercise and exposure to beautiful landscapes whilst bonding with horses! Whether trail riding through forested trails or galloping along sandy beaches - horseback riding offers an unforgettable experience! Consider taking lessons before heading out on your own as it's important not only for your safety but also the horse's wellbeing too!
- **Foraging -** Foraging is a unique way to explore nature while also discovering edible plants, berries, and mushrooms that can be used in meals. However, it's important to educate yourself on what's safe to eat before heading out into the wild. Consider taking a foraging class or hiring a guide to help you identify edible plants.
- **Hot Air Ballooning -** Hot air ballooning offers an incredible bird's eye view of nature, floating peacefully above forests, lakes & mountains! It's an exciting adventure that provides stunning panoramic views of landscapes whilst experiencing the thrill of being up high in the sky. Look for local hot air balloon companies that offer flights in your area!
- **Tree Climbing -** Tree climbing is a fun way to get active outdoors while also experiencing the beauty of trees from different angles! It's an excellent workout for both body & mind - requiring balance, focus & strength. Many communities have tree climbing groups or organizations that offer classes or guided climbs.

- **Camping -** Camping offers an opportunity to spend time immersed in nature by spending nights under the stars! Whether car camping in a national park or backpacking deep into wilderness areas - camping provides an escape from city life and allows one to fully unplug & recharge surrounded by natural beauty.

- **Paddleboarding -** Paddleboarding is another great water sport that allows you to explore lakes or oceans whilst standing on a board with a paddle! It provides both physical exercise and relaxation as you glide over calm waters whilst taking in natural surroundings such as wildlife & sunsets!

- **Disc Golf -** If you're looking for a new way to get outside and exercise, try disc golf! Similar to traditional golf, but instead of hitting a ball with a club, you throw Frisbee-like discs into baskets. It's a low-impact activity that can be enjoyed by people of all ages and skill levels.

- **Nature Photography -** Take your love for nature to the next level by trying out nature photography. Whether it's capturing a stunning landscape or photographing wildlife, there's always something new and exciting to discover through the lens of a camera.

- **Hiking -** Get some fresh air and exercise by taking up hiking! With endless trails to explore in national parks and forests, you'll never run out of new places to hike. Plus, hiking is a great way to stay fit and healthy during retirement.

- **Vegetable Gardening -** Start a vegetable garden in your backyard and enjoy the fruits (and vegetables) of your labor! Not only will gardening keep you active, but it's also a relaxing hobby that can provide fresh produce for healthy meals.

- **Beachcombing -** Spend some time at the beach searching for treasures washed ashore! From sea glass to shells and even fossils, beachcombing is a peaceful activity that allows you to connect with nature while enjoying the beauty of the ocean.

- **Outdoor Yoga -** Take your yoga practice outside and connect with nature! Whether it's in your backyard or at a local park, practicing yoga outdoors can be a peaceful and rejuvenating experience.

- **Orienteering -** Test your navigational skills by trying orienteering! Using only a map and compass, you'll navigate through an outdoor course filled with checkpoints along the way. It's a challenging yet rewarding activity that will keep you mentally sharp.

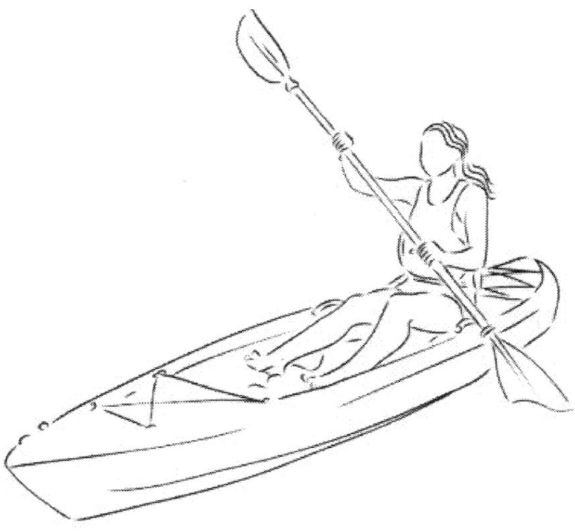

Solo Adventures

Remember, that retirement doesn't mean slowing down. In fact, it's the perfect time to try new things and explore your interests. Going solo can be a great way to challenge yourself and discover hidden tal-ents. In this chapter, we'll introduce you to a variety of activities that are perfect for those who want to enjoy their alone time while still making the most out of every day.

- **Geocaching** - Get ready for an adventure! Geocaching is like a modern-day treasure hunt using GPS coordinates. With millions of hidden caches all over the world, you can explore new places while searching for hidden treasures. It's a fun way to stay active and get in touch with nature.

- **Wilderness camping -** For those who love nature, wilderness camping is the ultimate adventure. Leave civilization behind and spend some time alone in the great outdoors. Just make sure you're prepared with all the necessary gear and safety precautions.

- **Volunteering abroad -** If you're looking for a more meaningful adventure, consider volunteering abroad. There are plenty of organizations that offer volunteer programs for retirees, from teaching English in Thailand to building homes in Guatemala. Not only will you get to experience a different culture, but you'll also be making a positive impact on the world.

- **Road tripping -** Hit the open road and explore your own country with a solo road trip. You can plan your route ahead of time or just go where the wind takes you. Take your time, stop at roadside attractions, and enjoy the freedom of traveling without an itinerary.

- **Learning a new skill -** Retirement is the perfect time to learn something new, whether it's painting, cooking, or even skydiving! Take a class or sign up for lessons and challenge yourself to try something outside of your comfort zone.
- **Urban exploration -** Explore the hidden gems of your city or a nearby metropolis by going on an urban adventure. Visit street art murals, abandoned buildings, and quirky shops you've never been to before. You can even create your own scavenger hunt to add an extra layer of excitement.
- **Bike touring -** If you love cycling, consider going on a solo bike tour. Plan out a route that takes you through scenic areas and interesting towns, and camp or stay in hostels along the way. It's a great way to challenge yourself physically while experiencing the beauty of nature.
- **Writing retreat -** For those who enjoy writing, consider taking a solo retreat to focus on your craft. Rent a cabin in the woods or a cozy apartment in the city where you can write without distractions. Use this time to work on that novel you've always wanted to write or simply journal about your retirement experiences.
- **Cultural immersion -** Immerse yourself in another culture by taking an extended trip abroad. Stay with locals through homestays or Airbnb rentals and learn about their customs and traditions firsthand. Take language classes or cooking lessons to deepen your understanding of the culture.

- **Outdoor fitness challenge -** Challenge yourself physically by setting an outdoor fitness goal like climbing a mountain or completing a long-distance hike. Train for it solo and then embark on the adventure alone – it will give you a sense of accomplishment and independence like no other!

- **Spiritual retreat -** Take a solo spiritual retreat to reconnect with yourself and your beliefs. Visit a monastery or ashram, attend a silent meditation retreat, or simply spend time in nature reflecting on your life's purpose.

- **Photography expedition -** If you love photography, take a solo trip to capture stunning shots of landscapes and cultures around the world. Plan out an itinerary that takes you to unique and picturesque locations and challenge yourself to capture the essence of each place through your lens.

- **House sitting -** Consider house sitting as a way to travel solo while also saving money on accommodation costs. There are many websites where homeowners post opportunities for house sitters to stay in their homes while they're away. This is a great way to experience local neighborhoods like a resident rather than a tourist.

- **Foodie adventures -** Embark on culinary adventures by exploring different cuisines from around the world or even taking cooking classes from renowned chefs. Try new dishes, attend food festivals, or even start your own food blog sharing your experiences with others.

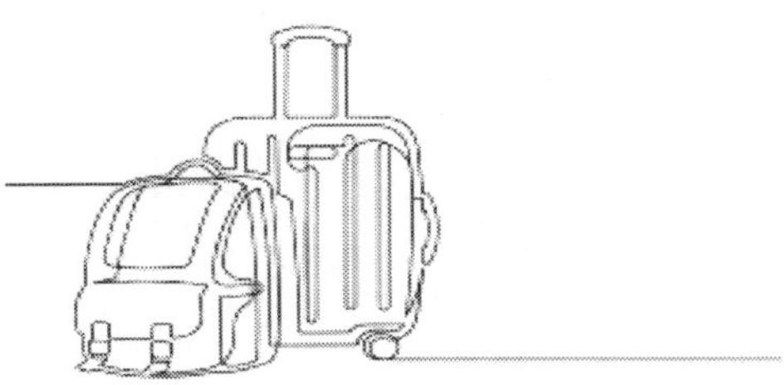

Exploring the Wonders of Water

It's time to explore the world around you! One way to do that is by experiencing the magic of water. In this chapter, we'll dive into some exciting aquatic adventures that will leave you feeling refreshed and invigorated. From peaceful kayaking trips to thrilling snorkeling excursions, there's something for everyone looking to make a splash in their retirement years. So grab your swimsuit and let's get started

- **Underwater Photography** - Take a dip with your camera and capture stunning images of marine life. Join a local photography club or take a specialized course to learn the ins and outs of underwater photography. You'll be amazed at the hidden beauty that lies beneath the surface.
- **Kayak Fishing** - Combine two popular water activities into one exciting adventure. Kayak fishing allows you to silently glide through calm waters while casting your line for a variety of fish species. It's a peaceful way to spend an afternoon on the water.
- **Mermaid Swimming** - Embrace your inner child and become a mermaid for a day! Mermaid swimming classes are becoming increasingly popular, offering adults the chance to don fins and learn how to swim with grace and elegance like our mythical counterparts.
- **Paddleboard Yoga** - Take your yoga practice outdoors by trying paddleboard yoga. Balancing on a paddleboard in the middle of the water adds an extra challenge to traditional yoga poses, making it both physically and mentally stimulating.

- **Snorkeling Tours** - Explore coral reefs and tropical fish habitats on guided snorkeling tours. Many tour companies offer excursions catered specifically towards retirees, allowing you to take in all the beauty without worrying about keeping up with younger participants.
- **Stand-Up Paddleboarding** - Stand-up paddleboarding (SUP) is a great way to enjoy the water while getting a full-body workout. It's easy to learn and can be done on calm lakes or even in the ocean waves.
- **Kayak Eco Tours** - Join a guided kayak tour through natural habitats like mangroves or estuaries. You'll learn about local ecosystems and wildlife while getting some exercise and fresh air.
- **White Water Rafting** - For the more adventurous retiree, white water rafting provides an adrenaline rush while navigating rapids with a team of fellow rafters. There are different levels of difficulty available, so you can choose one that suits your skill level.
- **Scuba Diving** - Take your underwater exploration to the next level by learning how to scuba dive. Many diving schools offer beginner courses that will teach you all the necessary skills and give you the chance to explore coral reefs and shipwrecks.
- **Sailing Lessons** - Always dreamed of sailing off into the sunset? Retirement is the perfect time to take sailing lessons and learn how to navigate open waters with confidence. Who knows, you may even decide to buy your own sailboat!

- **Jet Skiing** - For those who love speed and thrills, jet skiing is a great way to enjoy the water. Rent a jet ski and explore the coastline or participate in guided tours that take you to hidden coves and beaches.
- **Surfing Lessons** - Always wanted to ride the waves? Retirement is the perfect time to take up surfing lessons and learn how to catch waves like a pro. Many surf schools offer beginner courses that will teach you all the necessary skills.
- **Snuba Diving** - Snuba diving is a cross between snorkeling and scuba diving, allowing you to explore deeper waters without having to carry heavy equipment on your back. It's an exciting way to experience marine life up close.
- **Water Aerobics** - Water aerobics classes are a great way to stay active while enjoying the water. The buoyancy of the water reduces impact on joints, making it an ideal low-impact activity for retirees.
- **Whale Watching Tours** - Join a whale watching tour and witness these magnificent creatures in their natural habitat. Many tour companies offer excursions during peak whale watching seasons, giving you the chance to see humpback whales breach or killer whales hunt.

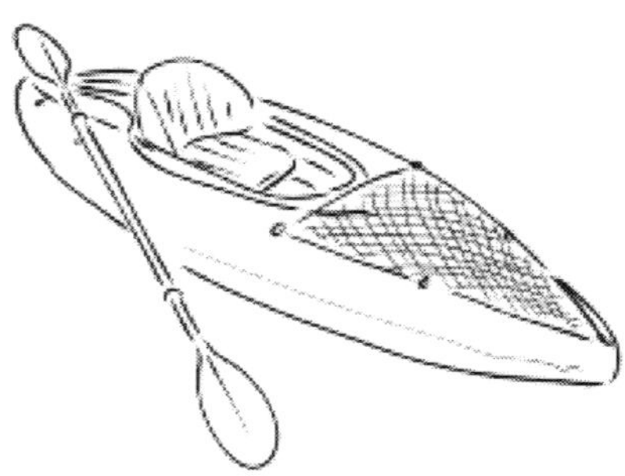

Relive Your Childhood Memories with Adult Summer Camps

Relive your childhood memories and make new ones by attending summer camps designed exclusively for adults. Engage in outdoor activities, learn new skills, and bond with like-minded individuals in a fun and nostalgic environment. From traditional camping experiences to specialized programs, there's something for everyone at adult summer camps.

- **Glamping -** Experience the great outdoors in style with glamping, or glamorous camping. Many summer camps for adults offer luxurious accommodations such as fully furnished tents, cabins, or even treehouses. Enjoy nature without sacrificing comfort.
- **Campfire Cooking Challenge -** Put your culinary skills to the test with a campfire cooking challenge. Gather ingredients from the surrounding wilderness and compete against fellow campers to create the most delicious meal over an open flame.
- **Adventure Races -** Get your adrenaline pumping with an adventure race at summer camp. These races can involve activities such as kayaking, rock climbing, and mountain biking, and are designed to challenge both physical and mental abilities.
- **Arts and Crafts Workshops -** Unleash your inner artist with arts and crafts workshops offered at many adult summer camps. Try your hand at pottery, painting, or jewelry making while surrounded by the natural beauty of your surroundings.

- **Stargazing Parties -** Take in the breathtaking night sky with stargazing parties hosted by experienced astronomers. Learn about constellations and planets while enjoying a peaceful evening under the stars.
- **Survival Skills Training -** Learn how to survive in the wilderness with survival skills training. From building a shelter to starting a fire without matches, these workshops will teach you how to thrive in nature.
- **Yoga and Meditation Retreats -** Find inner peace and relaxation with yoga and meditation retreats offered at many adult summer camps. Unwind with daily yoga classes and guided meditations while surrounded by the tranquility of nature.
- **Wine Tasting Tours -** Take a break from outdoor activities with wine tasting tours at local vineyards. Many adult summer camps offer transportation to nearby wineries for tastings and tours.
- **Team-Building Exercises -** Strengthen relationships and build teamwork skills with group exercises designed for team-building. These activities can include trust falls, problem-solving challenges, and communication exercises.
- **Dance Parties -** Let loose and have fun with dance parties held at summer camp. From line dancing to salsa lessons, there's something for everyone to enjoy on the dance floor.
- **Photography Workshops -** Learn how to capture the beauty of nature with photography workshops. Professional photographers will teach you techniques for taking stunning landscape photos and portraits in natural settings.

- **Bird-Watching Excursions -** Explore the diverse bird species that inhabit summer camp environments with guided bird-watching excursions. Learn about different bird calls and behaviors while enjoying a peaceful hike.

- **Outdoor Movie Nights -** Enjoy movie nights under the stars with outdoor screenings at adult summer camps. Snuggle up with blankets and popcorn while watching classic films on a large screen.

- **Creative Writing Workshops -** Unleash your creativity with writing workshops held at many adult summer camps. Hone your writing skills and get inspired by the natural surroundings to write poetry, short stories, or even a novel.

- **Eco-Tours -** Learn about sustainable living practices and environmental conservation efforts with eco-tours offered at some adult summer camps. Explore alternative energy sources, organic farming practices, and ways to reduce waste in everyday life.

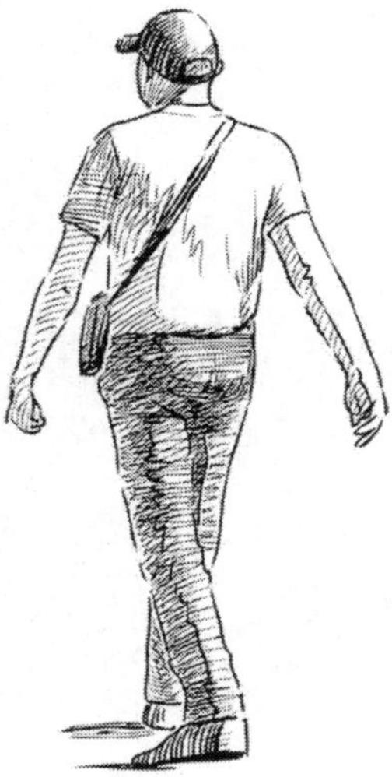

EXPLORING YOUR CREATIVE SIDE

Retirement is a time to explore new passions and hobbies, and what better way to do that than through artistic pursuits? Whether you are a seasoned artist or a beginner, this chapter will guide you through various creative activities that will not only keep your mind sharp but also bring joy and fulfillment to your life. From painting to pottery, from writing to music, there's something for everyone in this chapter. So let's dive in and discover the artist within you!

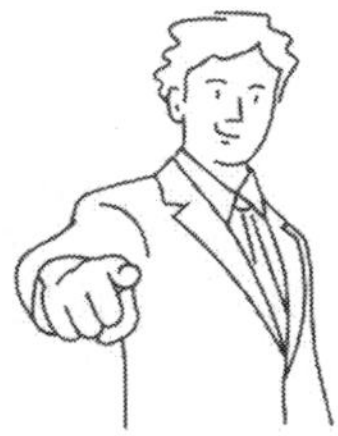

Fun and Fulfilling Crafts

Retirement is the perfect time to explore your creative side. In this chapter, we'll introduce you to a variety of hands-on activities that will keep your mind engaged and your hands busy. From knitting and painting to woodworking and pottery, there's something for everyone in the world of retirement crafts.

- **Paper Quilling** - Paper quilling is a fun and relaxing craft that involves rolling strips of paper into intricate designs. With just a few basic tools, you can create beautiful works of art that are perfect for decorating your home or giving as gifts.
- **Upcycling** - Upcycling is the practice of taking old, unwanted items and transforming them into something new and useful.

From turning an old sweater into a cozy throw pillow to repurposing a vintage suitcase into a stylish end table, the possibilities are endless.

- **Mosaic Art** - Mosaic art involves creating images by arranging small pieces of colored glass, ceramic tile, or other materials. It's a great way to express yourself creatively while also making something beautiful for your home or garden.
- **Felting** - Felting is a process that involves matting wool fibers together to create a dense fabric. With just some wool roving, soap, water, and elbow grease, you can make everything from cozy slippers to decorative wall hangings.
- **Embroidery** - Embroidery is an age-old craft that involves stitching designs onto fabric using colorful thread. From adding a personal touch to clothing and accessories to creating one-of-a-kind wall art, embroidery is a versatile and rewarding hobby that's perfect for retirees looking for something fun and creative to do in their free time.
- **Candle Making** - Candle making is a relaxing and creative hobby that allows you to make beautiful candles in different shapes, sizes, and colors. You can customize the scent and texture of your candles to suit your preferences.
- **Macrame** - Macrame is the art of knotting cord or string in patterns to create decorative items such as wall hangings, plant hangers, and jewelry. It's a simple yet satisfying craft that requires only a few basic supplies.
- **Woodworking** - Woodworking is a versatile craft that allows you to create functional pieces such as furniture, shelves, and

picture frames. With some basic tools and materials, you can unleash your creativity and build something unique.

- **Soap Making** - Soap making is a fun way to create personalized soaps using natural ingredients like essential oils, herbs, and flowers. You can experiment with different scents, textures, and colors to make soap bars that are perfect for your skin type.
- **Jewelry Making** - Jewelry making is a rewarding hobby that enables you to create unique pieces of jewelry using beads, wire, metals, and stones. You can design necklaces, bracelets or earrings to match any outfit or occasion.
- **Calligraphy** - Calligraphy is the art of writing beautifully using a pen or brush. It's a relaxing and meditative craft that can be used to create stunning invitations, cards, and wall art.
- **Knitting or Crocheting** - Knitting or crocheting is a classic craft that allows you to create cozy and warm items such as scarves, hats, blankets, and sweaters. It's a satisfying hobby that helps improve dexterity and concentration.
- **Paint Pouring** - Paint pouring is an abstract art technique that involves pouring acrylic paint onto a canvas to create unique patterns and textures. It's an easy yet impressive way to make beautiful pieces of art.
- **Pottery** - Pottery is a therapeutic craft that allows you to create functional items such as bowls, mugs, vases, and plates using clay. You can experiment with different shapes, textures, and glazes to make something truly unique.

- **Sewing** - Sewing is a practical skill that enables you to create clothing, home decor items like curtains or tablecloths or repair worn-out garments in your wardrobe. You can choose from various fabric options and styles based on your preferences.

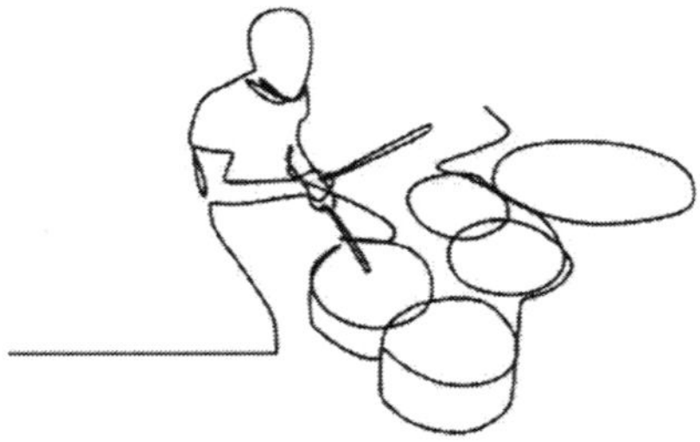

Get Creative in Your Personal Oasis

Find new and exciting ways to fi ll your newfound free time. One of the simplest yet most fulfi lling ways to do this is by heading out to your shed. In this chapter, we'll explore a variety of activities that can be done in your shed, providing both practical and creative outlets for your newfound leisure time.

- **Shed Organization Challenge -** Spend a day decluttering and organizing your shed. Not only will it help you find what you need more easily, but it will also give you a sense of accomplishment.

- **Greenhouse Gardening -** Turn your shed into a greenhouse and start growing your own fruits, vegetables, and flowers. It's a great way to stay active and create something beautiful at the same time.

- **DIY Woodworking Projects -** If you're handy with tools, try your hand at some DIY woodworking projects in your shed. Build birdhouses, bookshelves, or even furniture for your home.

- **Meditation Space -** Transform your shed into a peaceful retreat where you can practice meditation or yoga. Add some comfortable seating and calming decor to create an oasis of tranquility.

- **Home Brewery -** Always dreamed of brewing your own beer? With the right equipment and supplies, you can turn your shed into a home brewery and start experimenting with different recipes.

- **Art Studio -** Set up an art studio in your shed and explore your creative side. Paint, draw, or sculpt to your heart's content, and enjoy the freedom of expression that comes with retirement.

- **Music Room -** If you're a musician, turn your shed into a music room where you can practice and record music. Soundproofing is key here, so invest in some quality insulation to keep the noise from disturbing your neighbors.

- **Home Theater -** Create a cozy home theater in your shed by adding comfortable seating, a big screen TV, and surround sound speakers. It's a great way to enjoy movies and shows without leaving the comfort of your own home.

- **Indoor Golf Simulator -** Love golf but don't want to brave the elements? Turn your shed into an indoor golf simulator with a putting green, netting, and virtual reality technology that lets you play on some of the world's best courses.

- **Beekeeping -** If you're interested in beekeeping, turn your shed into a hive where you can raise bees and harvest honey. Not only is it fun and rewarding, but it also helps support local ecosystems by promoting pollination.

- **Photography Studio -** Turn your shed into a photography studio where you can experiment with different lighting, backdrops, and props. It's a great way to capture memories and express your artistic vision.
- **Pottery Studio -** Get your hands dirty by turning your shed into a pottery studio. Invest in a wheel, kiln, and clay supplies to create beautiful ceramics that you can use or give as gifts.
- **Writing Room -** If you're an aspiring writer, turn your shed into a writing room where you can work on your craft in peace and quiet. Add some comfortable seating, a desk, and some inspiration quotes to get the creative juices flowing.
- **DIY Car Repair Shop -** If you're handy with cars, turn your shed into a DIY car repair shop where you can work on your own vehicles or help friends and family with theirs.
- **Animal Shelter -** If you love animals, consider turning your shed into an animal shelter for rescued cats or dogs. Work with local animal welfare organizations to provide care for animals in need while enjoying their company yourself.

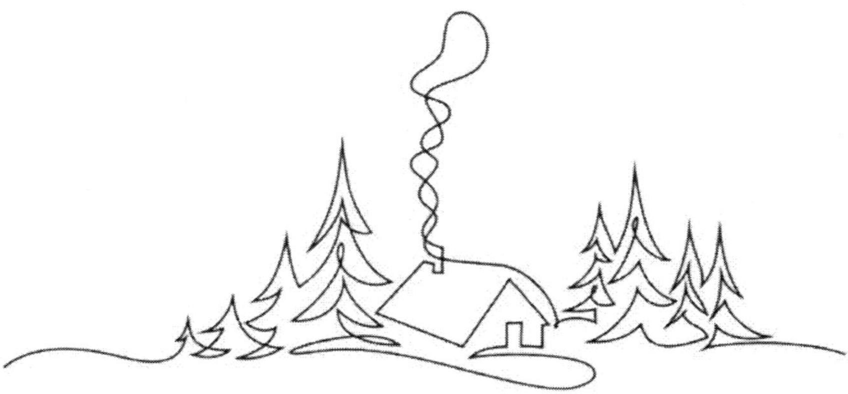

Creating a Fulfilling Social Life

Maintain social connections and cultivate new ones. In this chapter, we'll explore ways to stay connected with friends and family while also branch-ing out and meeting new people. From group activities to solo ad-ventures, there's something for everyone looking to maintain an active social life in retirement.

- **Volunteer at a local animal shelter -** Spend your free time cuddling and playing with furry friends while giving back to your community. Not only will you be helping animals in need, but you'll also meet other like-minded volunteers who share your love for animals.
- **Join a local theater group -** Always dreamed of being an actor? Retirement is the perfect time to pursue that dream! Joining a local theater group is a great way to meet new people, learn new skills, and have fun performing on stage.
- **Attend a murder mystery dinner party -** Put your detective skills to the test by attending a murder mystery dinner party! These events typically involve solving a fictional crime while enjoying dinner and drinks with other guests. It's a fun way to socialize and use your brain at the same time.
- **Host a potluck game night -** Invite friends over for a potluck game night! Everyone brings their favorite dish and board game, and you spend the evening eating, laughing, and having fun together.

- **Join a book club -** Reading is a great way to stimulate your mind and engage with others. Consider joining a local book club or starting one of your own. You'll get to read interesting books, discuss them with others, and make new friends along the way.

- **Take a cooking class -** Always wanted to learn how to cook Thai food? Retirement is the perfect time to take that cooking class you've been dreaming of. Not only will you learn a new skill, but you'll also have the opportunity to meet other foodies who share your passion for culinary delights.

- **Attend a wine tasting event -** If you're a wine enthusiast, attending a wine tasting event can be a great social activity. You'll get to sample different wines, learn about their origins and flavors, and connect with other wine lovers in your area.

- **Learn a new language -** Learning a new language is not only good for your brain but it's also an excellent way to meet new people from different cultures. Consider taking language classes at your local community college or using online resources like Duolingo or Rosetta Stone.

- **Join a hiking group -** Hiking is not only great exercise but it's also an excellent way to explore nature and connect with others who enjoy the outdoors. Joining a hiking group in your area can help you discover new trails while making friends along the way.

- **Attend a paint and sip event -** These events typically involve painting a picture while enjoying a glass of wine or other beverage. It's a fun way to get creative and socialize with others who share your love of art.

- **Join a local choir or singing group -** If you enjoy singing, joining a local choir or singing group can be a great way to connect with others who share your passion for music. You'll get to practice and perform together while making new friends along the way.
- **Take up ballroom dancing -** Ballroom dancing is not only great exercise but it's also an excellent way to socialize and meet new people. Consider taking classes at your local community center or dance studio.
- **Attend a comedy club -** Laughter is the best medicine, so why not attend a comedy club with friends? You'll get to enjoy stand-up comedy while bonding over shared laughs.
- **Participate in a community service project -** Volunteering for community service projects is not only fulfilling but it's also an excellent way to meet new people who share your values. Consider participating in projects like cleaning up local parks or helping out at food banks.

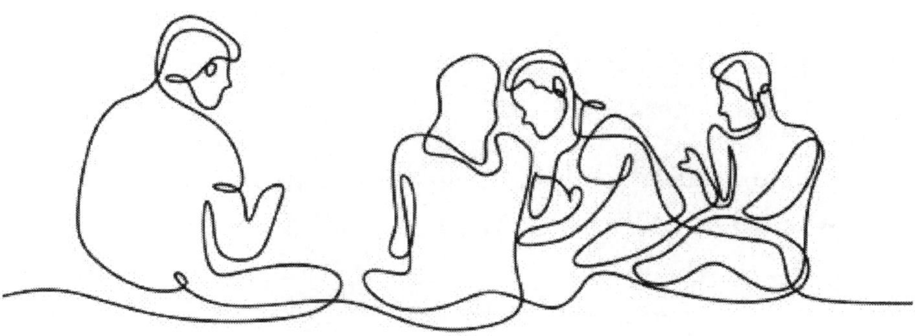

The Power of Music

Retirement is the perfect time to explore new hobbies and interests, and music is a great way to do just that. Whether you've always wanted to learn an instrument or just enjoy listening to live performances, this chapter offers a variety of musical activities to keep you entertained and engaged in your retirement years. From attending local concerts to joining a community choir, there's something for everyone in the world of retirement music.

- **Songwriting -** Have you ever wanted to express yourself through music? Retirement is the perfect time to give songwriting a try. Spend an afternoon writing lyrics or composing a melody. You may be surprised at what you come up with! Not only is songwriting a creative outlet, but it can also be therapeutic.

- **Garage Band -** Gather some friends who share your love of music and form your own garage band. Even if you've never played an instrument before, there are plenty of beginner-friendly instruments like ukuleles or bongos that can get you started on the path to rock stardom! Rehearsing with friends is not only fun but also provides social interaction and keeps you mentally sharp.

- **Attend a Music Festival -** Retirement is the perfect time to attend a music festival like Coachella or Bonnaroo. These festivals offer a wide variety of genres and provide an opportunity to see live performances from some of the biggest names in music as well as discover new artists.

- **Musical Theater -** Join a local theater group or audition for community productions of popular musicals like Hamilton, The Lion King, or Les Miserables. It's never too late to start acting or singing, and participating in musical theater provides an opportunity for self-expression while also keeping your mind active.
- **Learn a New Instrument -** Always wanted to learn how to play the guitar or piano? Retirement offers ample time for pursuing such interests! Sign up for lessons at a local music school or hire a private instructor for one-on-one instruction tailored specifically for seniors.
- **Karaoke Night -** Gather some friends for a fun night of karaoke singing. Many bars and restaurants offer karaoke nights where you can take turns belting out your favorite tunes. It's a great way to let loose and have fun while also improving your vocal skills.
- **Music Therapy -** Consider enrolling in music therapy sessions to improve mental health and well-being. Music therapy has been shown to be effective in reducing stress, anxiety, and depression, as well as improving cognitive function in older adults.
- **Attend a Symphony or Opera -** Retirement offers the perfect opportunity to indulge in cultural experiences like attending a symphony or opera performance. Check local listings for upcoming shows that may interest you and enjoy an evening out on the town.

- **Volunteer with Local Music Programs -** Many schools and community centers offer music programs for children or underserved populations that could benefit from volunteer support. Consider volunteering your time to help teach music classes or assist with performances.

- **Record Your Own Album -** If you're feeling ambitious, why not record your own album? With modern technology, it's easier than ever to create professional-quality recordings from the comfort of your own home studio. Whether it's covers of your favorite songs or original compositions, recording an album is a rewarding accomplishment that can be shared with family and friends.

- **Attend Music Conferences -** Retirement is a great time to attend music conferences and workshops where you can learn more about the industry, network with other musicians and professionals, and improve your skills. Look for events that cater to your interests, whether it's songwriting, music production or performance.

- **Join a Choir -** Joining a choir is a great way to stay active musically while also meeting new people in your community. Many choirs welcome senior members and offer regular performances throughout the year.

- **Create a Music Playlist -** Spend some time creating a music playlist that reflects your personal tastes and preferences. You can use online streaming services like Spotify or Apple Music to curate your own playlists or explore curated playlists based on different genres or themes.

- **Learn About Music History -** Retirement provides ample time for learning new things, so why not dive into the history of music? There are many books, documentaries, podcasts and online courses that explore the evolution of music through the ages.
- **Write Musical Reviews -** If you enjoy attending concerts or listening to new albums, consider writing reviews of the performances or recordings you experience. You can share these reviews on social media platforms like Facebook or Instagram or start your own blog where you can publish your thoughts on various musical topics.

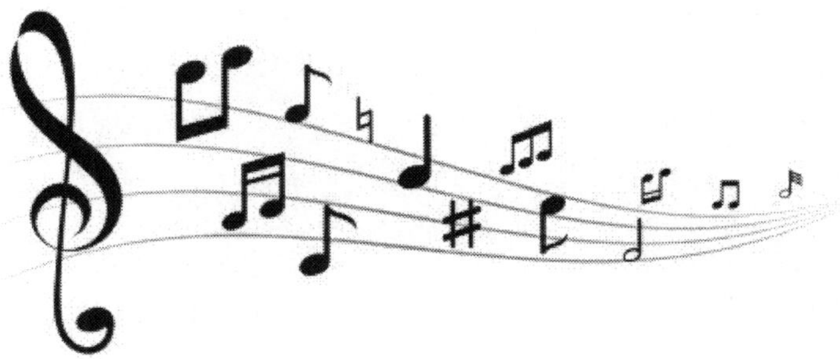

Unlocking Your Creative Potential

Keep your mind sharp and your creativity flowing. In this chapter, we will explore a variety of activities that will inspire you to tap into your inner artist, from painting and photography to writing and even acting. Whether you're a seasoned pro or a beginner, these activities are sure to provide endless hours of enjoyment and fulfillment in your retirement years.

- **Artistic Journaling -** Start an artistic journal where you can jot down your thoughts, dreams, and experiences in a creative way. Use different colors, textures, stickers, and images to make each entry unique.
- **Poetry Writing -** Get in touch with your inner poet by writing haikus or free verse poems about anything that inspires you. Share them with friends and family or even submit them to literary magazines for publication.
- **Photography Walks -** Take regular walks with your camera in hand and capture the beauty of nature around you. Experiment with different angles, lighting, and settings to create stunning photographs that showcase your unique perspective on the world.
- **Creative Writing -** Explore your imagination by writing short stories or even a novel. Join a writing group or take an online class to hone your skills and receive feedback on your work.
- **Music Lessons -** Learn to play an instrument or take singing lessons to express yourself through music. You could even start a band with other retired musicians in your community!

- **Scrapbooking -** Create scrapbooks of your travels, family memories, or hobbies. Use colorful paper, stickers, and embellishments to make each page unique and reflective of your personality.
- **Gardening -** Cultivate a garden that reflects your creativity and personal style. Experiment with different plants, flowers, and landscaping techniques to create a beautiful outdoor space.
- **Crafting -** Try out various crafting techniques such as knitting, crocheting, quilting, or woodworking. Create handmade gifts for loved ones or even sell your creations at local craft fairs.
- **Acting -** Join a local theater group or take acting classes to explore your dramatic side. You could even audition for community theater productions or participate in improv comedy groups.
- **Film Critique -** Start a film critique club with friends where you watch and review films together. Analyze the cinematography, character development, and storyline while expressing your opinions and thoughts about each movie.
- **Stand-Up Comedy -** Take a stand-up comedy class or workshop to learn how to write and perform your own jokes. Try out your material at open mic nights or even start performing professionally!
- **Creative Dance -** Take dance classes such as ballet, jazz, contemporary, or hip-hop to express yourself through movement. Join a local dance troupe or just dance for pleasure in the comfort of your own home.

- **Volunteer Work -** Volunteer for organizations that allow you to express your creativity while making a difference in the community. Examples include teaching art classes at a senior center, designing flyers for a charity event, or creating costumes for a local theater production.

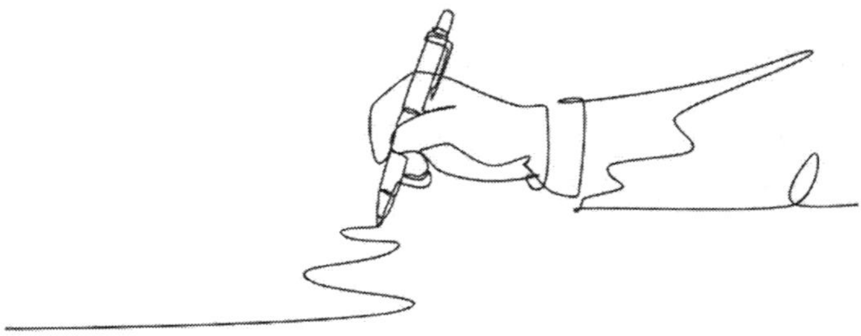

Cultivating your Dream Garden

Time to find new ways to stay active and engaged. Gardening is a wonderful hobby that not only keeps us physically active but also provides a sense of purpose and accomplishment. In this chapter, we will explore vari-ous gardening activities that can bring beauty and life to your out-door space while also providing a fulfi lling pastime.

- **Seed Bombing** - Create small balls of soil mixed with seeds and throw them in abandoned lots, roadside areas or any place that needs some greenery. Watch as wildflowers and other plants sprout up from your seed bombs.

- **Fairy Garden** - Create a miniature garden filled with tiny plants, stones, and figurines to create an enchanted world for fairies or other magical creatures.

- **Vertical Gardening** - If you have limited space, try growing plants vertically on walls or fences using trellises or hanging baskets.
- **Hypertufa Planters** - Make your own rustic-looking planters out of hypertufa – a mixture of cement, peat moss, and perlite – that resembles stone but is much lighter.
- **Espalier Fruit Trees** - Train fruit trees to grow flat against walls or fences in decorative patterns like diamonds or squares to save space and add visual interest to your garden.
- **Herb Spiral** - Create a spiral-shaped garden bed using bricks, stones or other materials and plant herbs in each section. This design maximizes space and allows for easy access to all plants.
- **Succulent Wall Art** - Create living wall art by attaching succulents to a wooden frame or pallet. This low-maintenance project adds a unique touch to any outdoor space.
- **Beekeeping** - Start your own beehive and help support the declining bee population while enjoying fresh honey and beeswax products.
- **Garden Yoga** - Practice yoga in your garden surrounded by nature's beauty. Use garden benches, trees, and other props for support during poses.
- **Garden Art Projects** - Add some personality to your garden with unique art projects such as birdhouses, stepping stones, or mosaic tiles made from broken pottery or glass.

- **Aquaponics** - Combine fish farming and gardening by creating a closed-loop system where fish waste fertilizes plants and plants filter the water for the fish.
- **Garden Photography** - Capture the beauty of your garden with photography. Experiment with different angles, lighting, and lenses to create stunning shots.
- **Terrariums** - Create miniature ecosystems in glass containers filled with soil, rocks, and small plants. These low-maintenance gardens add a unique touch to any indoor space.
- **Garden Sculptures** - Add some art to your garden with sculptures made from natural materials such as driftwood or stones.
- **Rainwater Harvesting** - Collect rainwater in barrels or other containers to use for watering plants during dry spells.

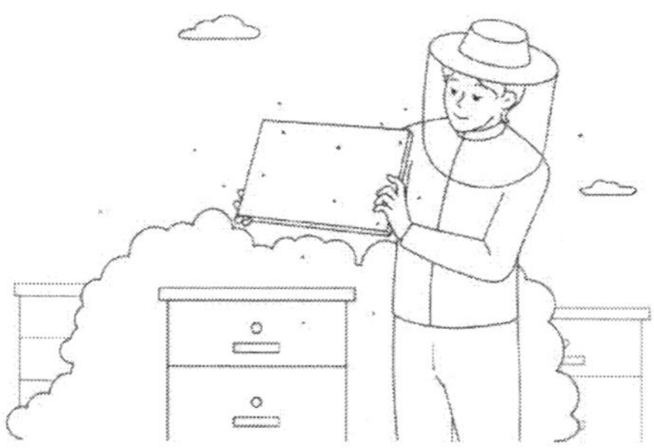

The Fun of Making Things

Retirement is the perfect time to explore your creative side and engage in activities that bring you joy. In this chapter, we'll dive into the world of making things by exploring fantastic hobbies such as soap making and carving. Whether you're a seasoned crafter or just starting out, these activities are sure to bring a sense of fulfillment and satisfaction to your retirement years. So grab your tools and let's get started!

- **DIY Herb Garden -** Create your own herb garden by repurposing old wooden pallets. With a little sanding and staining, you can transform a pallet into a beautiful planter for your favorite herbs. Not only will you have fresh herbs at your fingertips, but you'll also enjoy the satisfaction of creating something useful from scratch.

- **Upcycled Jewelry -** Turn old broken jewelry or thrift store finds into one-of-a-kind accessories. Use pliers and wire cutters to take apart pieces, then reassemble them in new ways or add beads or charms for a personal touch. You'll love wearing jewelry that's both eco-friendly and uniquely yours.

- **Handmade Soap -** Crafting soap is easier than you might think! All it takes is some basic ingredients like coconut oil, lye, and essential oils to create bars that smell amazing and are gentle on skin. Plus, you can experiment with different colors and shapes to make them truly unique.

- **Knitting or Crocheting -** These classic hobbies are perfect for retirement because they're portable and relaxing yet still provide a sense of accomplishment when completed projects are displayed or given as gifts. Start with simple scarves or dishcloths before moving on to more complex patterns like sweaters or blankets.

- **Paper Crafts -** From origami to scrapbooking, paper crafts offer endless possibilities for creativity. Create personalized cards or invitations, make decorations for holidays or special events or even try making 3D paper sculptures.

- **Soapstone Carving -** Discover the ancient art of carving soapstone into beautiful sculptures or functional objects like bowls and vases. With some basic tools and techniques, you can unleash your inner artist and create something truly unique and timeless.
- **Glassblowing -** Try your hand at glassblowing and create unique, colorful pieces like vases, bowls or even ornaments. With some basic equipment and the guidance of an experienced instructor, you can create beautiful glass objects that will impress everyone who sees them.
- **Leatherworking -** Learn how to work with leather to create custom belts, wallets or even shoes. With a few basic tools and some quality leather, you can craft functional items that are both stylish and long-lasting.
- **Wood Carving -** Take up the timeless craft of wood carving and make intricate designs in everything from walking sticks to figurines. With a bit of patience and practice, you can create stunning works of art that showcase your creativity and skill.
- **Metalworking -** Learn how to weld or solder metal to make sculptures, jewelry or even furniture. This versatile medium offers endless possibilities for creativity and can be used to create durable pieces that will last for generations.

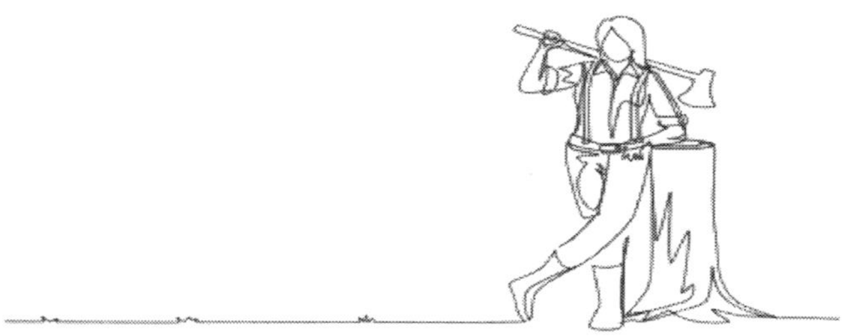

LIFELONG LEARNING DURING RETIREMENT

Retirement is a time to explore new things, learn new skills, and broaden your horizons. In this chapter, we'll explore some of the best educational activities that will keep your mind sharp and engaged during your first year of retirement. From taking classes at local community colleges to attending lectures by renowned experts in various fields, there are countless opportunities for you to continue learning and growing in retirement. So why not make this year unforgettable by embarking on some exciting educational endeavors?

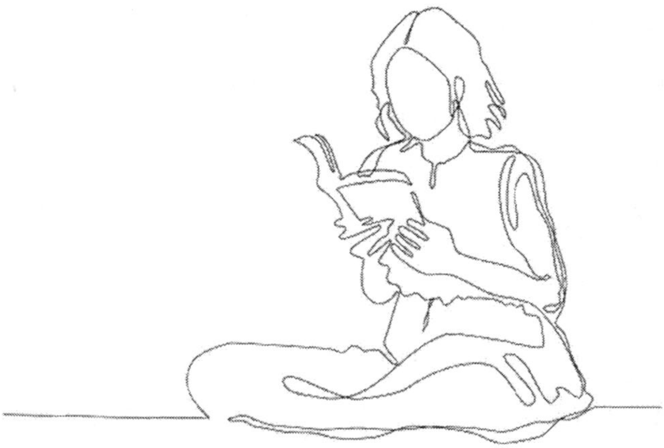

Expanding Your Horizons: Discovering New Passions

Continue challenging yourself and expanding your horizons. Learning a new skill can not only provide a sense of accomplishment but also keep your mind sharp. In this chapter, we'll explore various activities that will allow you to try something new and potentially discover a hidden talent.

- **Glassblowing -** Have you ever watched a glassblower at work and been mesmerized by their skill? Why not try it out for yourself? Many studios offer classes for beginners, where you can learn the basics of shaping and blowing glass.
- **Carpentry -** Always wanted to build your own furniture or fix up your home? Carpentry is a useful skill that can save you money in the long run. Take a class at your local community college or find online tutorials to get started.
- **Soap-making -** Making soap can be both practical and fun! You'll have control over what ingredients go into your soap, which means you can avoid harsh chemicals found in many store-bought brands. There are many recipes available online, so start experimenting with different scents and textures today!
- **Archery -** Channel your inner Robin Hood by taking up archery! It's a great way to improve your focus and hand-eye coordination. Find a local archery club or range that offers lessons for beginners.
- **Stand-up Comedy -** Always been the life of the party? Why not try your hand at stand-up comedy? Many cities offer open mic nights where you can test out your material in front of a live audience.
- **Calligraphy -** The art of calligraphy involves beautiful handwriting and lettering. It can be a relaxing and meditative hobby, perfect for retirement. Start with basic supplies like pens, ink, and paper, and find online tutorials to help you get started.

- **Wine-making -** Have you ever wanted to make your own wine? Retirement is the perfect time to learn this skill! You'll need some basic equipment such as carboys, corks, and bottles, but there are many kits available online that make it easy for beginners to get started. Cheers!

- **Bookbinding -** Bookbinding is the art of creating handmade books. It can be a relaxing and meditative hobby, perfect for retirement. Start with basic supplies like paper, glue, and thread, and find online tutorials to help you get started.

- **Photography -** Always had an eye for capturing beautiful moments? Why not take up photography as a hobby? You'll need a camera and some basic equipment, but there are many online tutorials available to help you develop your skills.

- **Dancing -** Whether it's ballroom dancing or hip hop, learning how to dance is a great way to stay active while also having fun! Find local dance classes or join a dance group in your community.

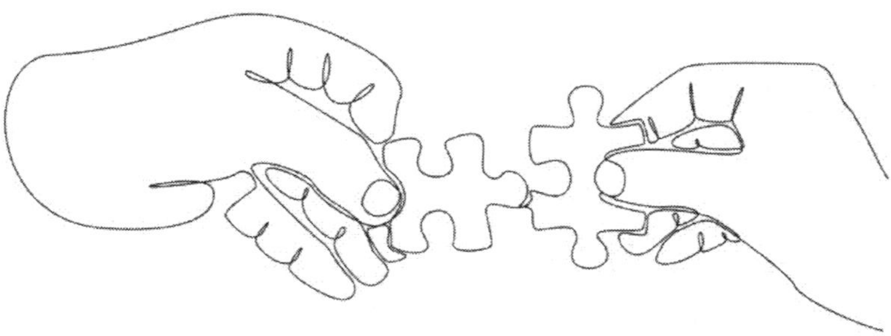

Discovering Your Family History

In this chapter, we delve into the fascinating world of your family history. Discovering where we come from and the stories of our ancestors can be a deeply enriching experience. From tracing your family tree to visiting ancestral homes, there are many ways to connect with your past and gain a greater understanding of your heritage.

- **Genealogy Road Trip -** Plan a road trip to visit the places where your ancestors lived, worked, and played. Take photos and document your journey, then create a scrapbook or blog post to share with your family.
- **Family Recipe Swap -** Gather recipes from your extended family members and compile them into a cookbook or online recipe collection. Make some of the dishes together and share stories about the origins of each recipe.
- **Cemetery Scavenger Hunt -** Visit local cemeteries and search for gravesites of your ancestors. Use online resources like FindAGrave.com to locate specific headstones, then take rubbings or leave flowers as a tribute.
- **Oral History Interviews -** Record interviews with older relatives to capture their memories of growing up, family traditions, and significant events in their lives. These recordings can be preserved for future generations to enjoy.
- **Heritage Crafts -** Learn traditional crafts that were practiced by your ancestors, such as quilting, weaving, or woodworking. Attend workshops or classes in these skills to connect with

others who share an interest in preserving cultural heritage through the arts.

- **Virtual Museum Tour -** Take a virtual tour of museums that showcase the culture and traditions of your family's heritage. Many museums offer online exhibits, videos, and interactive displays that can provide a wealth of information.
- **Family Tree Wall Art -** Create a unique piece of art by designing a family tree wall hanging or mural. Use photos, memorabilia, and other decorative elements to make it a special tribute to your family's history.
- **Ancestral Home Renovation -** If you have the resources and inclination, consider renovating or restoring an ancestral home or building. This can be a meaningful way to preserve your family's legacy while also creating a new living space for yourself.
- **Cultural Immersion Travel -** Plan a trip to the country or region where your ancestors originated from. Immerse yourself in the local culture by attending festivals, trying traditional foods, and visiting historical sites related to your family's heritage.
- **Storytelling Circle -** Host a storytelling circle with members of your extended family, where everyone shares their favorite memories or stories about relatives who have passed away. This can be a heartwarming way to connect with loved ones and keep cherished memories alive for future generations.
- **DNA Testing -** Take a DNA test to uncover your ethnic background and connect with relatives you may not have known existed. This can be a fascinating way to learn more about your

family's history and potentially discover new branches of your family tree.

- **Family History Book Club -** Start a book club with friends or family members where you read and discuss books related to genealogy, family history, or cultural traditions. This can provide opportunities for lively discussions and sharing of personal stories.

- **Heirloom Preservation -** If you have family heirlooms such as jewelry, furniture, or artwork, consider restoring or preserving them for future generations to enjoy. You can also create a catalog or online gallery of these items along with their histories.

- **Historical Reenactments -** Participate in historical reenactments that recreate events from your family's past such as battles, migrations, or cultural celebrations. This can be a fun way to experience history firsthand while also connecting with others who share your interests.

- **Cultural Exchange -** Host an exchange student from the country where your ancestors originated from or volunteer with organizations that promote cross-cultural understanding. This can be a meaningful way to learn more about your heritage while also fostering global connections.

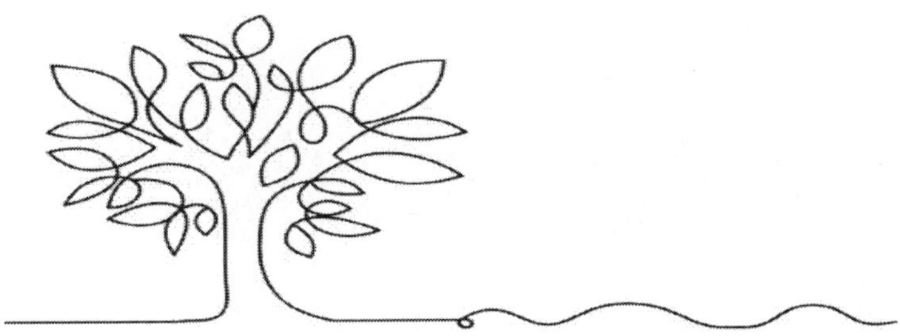

Technical Pursuits

Let us explore exciting activities that will challenge your mind and keep you engaged during your retirement. Whether it's learning how to code, mastering a new software program, or delving into the world of robotics, these pursuits will push you to learn new skills and expand your knowledge base. Get ready to embrace the technical side of life and discover a whole new world of possibilities!

- **Build Your Own Computer -** If you've ever been interested in how computers work, building your own can be a fun and rewarding experience. There are plenty of online tutorials and guides available that can walk you through the process step by step, and once you're finished, you'll have a custom computer that's tailored to your exact needs.

- **Learn Coding -** With so much of our lives now taking place online, knowing how to code can be an incredibly valuable skill. There are many free resources available online that can teach you everything from basic HTML and CSS to more advanced programming languages like Python or Java.

- **Dabble in Electronics -** Whether it's building your own custom sound system or creating your own home automation system, dabbling in electronics can be a fun and challenging pursuit. There are plenty of DIY kits available online that can help get you started, or if you're feeling ambitious, you could try designing your own circuits from scratch.

- **Try 3D Printing -** 3D printing has revolutionized the way we think about manufacturing, and now it's easier than ever to get started with this exciting technology. Whether you want to create custom jewelry or design your own toys, there are plenty of affordable 3D printers on the market that are perfect for home use.

- **Explore Virtual Reality -** Virtual reality is quickly becoming one of the most exciting new technologies on the market, and retirement is the perfect time to dive in and explore all that it has to offer. From gaming to education to virtual travel experiences, there's something for everyone in this rapidly growing field.

- **Learn Graphic Design -** Whether you want to create custom designs for your own personal projects or help out friends and family with their design needs, learning graphic design can be a fun and rewarding skill to have. There are many online tutorials and courses available that can teach you the basics of graphic design software like Adobe Photoshop or Illustrator.

- **Explore Robotics -** If you're interested in engineering or mechanics, exploring robotics can be an exciting new pursuit during retirement. From building your own robots from scratch to programming them to perform specific tasks, there are many ways to get involved in this fascinating field.

- **Try App Development -** With so many people relying on smartphones and tablets for their daily needs, app development has become an incredibly popular field in recent years. Whether you want to create a simple game or a productivity app that helps people stay organized, there are plenty of resources available online that can help you get started.

- **Experiment with Augmented Reality -** Augmented reality is another exciting new technology that's quickly gaining popularity across a wide range of industries. From creating your own augmented reality experiences using tools like ARKit or ARCore to exploring existing apps and experiences, there's no shortage of opportunities to get involved in this cutting-edge field.

- **Dive into Data Science -** With so much data being generated every day, understanding how to analyze and interpret it can be an incredibly valuable skill in today's job market. Whether you're interested in business analytics, machine learning, or data visualization, there are many online courses and resources available that can help you develop these skills.

- **Explore Cybersecurity -** As technology continues to advance, cybersecurity has become an increasingly important field. Learning how to protect yourself and others from online threats can be a valuable and rewarding pursuit during retirement. There are many online courses and resources available that can teach you the basics of cybersecurity and help you stay safe online.

- **Try your hand at Photography -** With the rise of digital cameras and smartphones, photography has become an incredibly popular hobby in recent years. Whether you're interested in landscape photography, portrait photography, or something in between, there are many tutorials and resources available that can help you improve your skills.

- **Learn Video Editing -** Whether you want to create your own YouTube channel or just edit family videos for fun, learning video editing can be a fun and rewarding skill to have. There are many free video editing software options available online that can help get you started.

- **Experiment with Virtual Assistants -** From Amazon's Alexa to Google Assistant, virtual assistants have become an increasingly popular way to interact with technology in our daily lives. Experimenting with different virtual assistants during retirement can be a fun way to learn about new technologies and find new ways to streamline your daily routine.

- **Build Your Own Website -** Whether it's for personal or professional use, building your own website can be a fulfilling project during retirement. There are many free website builders available online that make it easy to design and launch your own custom site without any coding knowledge required.

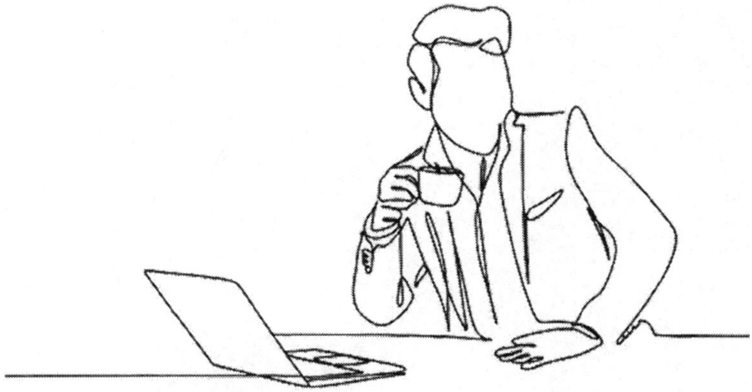

LEAVE A LASTING LEGACY

Retirement is not just about relaxing and taking it easy. It's also a time to give back to the community that has been an important part of your life for so many years. In this chapter, we'll explore different ways you can make a positive impact in your community and find fulfillment through volunteering and charitable work. From mentoring young people to helping out at a local food bank, there are countless opportunities to make a difference and leave a lasting legacy in your retirement years. Let's dive in and discover how you can give back while enjoying all the benefits of your newfound freedom!

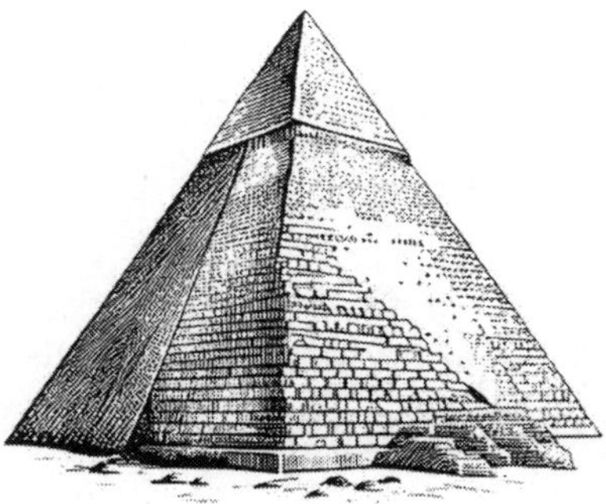

Making a Difference by Donating Your Time

In this chapter, we explore the fulfilling experience of donating your time during retirement. Giving back to the community not only benefits those in need but also provides a sense of purpose and satisfaction for retirees. Discover various volunteer opportunities that align with your interests and skills, and make a positive impact on the world around you.

- **Pet Therapy -** Spend time with furry friends in need of love and attention at your local animal shelter. Not only will you brighten their day, but studies have shown that interacting with animals can reduce stress and improve overall well-being.

- **Volunteer Abroad -** Combine travel with philanthropy by volunteering abroad with organizations like Global Volunteers or Habitat for Humanity. You'll get to experience new cultures while making a meaningful impact on communities in need.
- **Teach Adult Education Classes -** Share your expertise and skills by teaching adult education classes at your local community center or library. From cooking to woodworking, there's always someone eager to learn something new.
- **Virtual Volunteering -** Use technology to give back from the comfort of your own home through virtual volunteering opportunities such as online tutoring, writing letters to seniors, or transcribing historical documents for archives.
- **Disaster Relief -** Join disaster relief organizations like the Red Cross or Team Rubicon and help those affected by natural disasters rebuild their lives. Your physical labor and emotional support can make all the difference during a difficult time.
- **Mentorship -** Share your knowledge and experience with the next generation by becoming a mentor. You can volunteer with organizations like Big Brothers Big Sisters or mentor students at your local school.
- **Environmental Conservation -** Get involved in preserving our planet by volunteering with environmental conservation organizations like The Nature Conservancy or Sierra Club. You can help protect natural habitats, clean up parks and beaches, and plant trees to combat deforestation.
- **Hospital Volunteer -** Spread joy and support patients by volunteering at your local hospital. You can assist with tasks like

delivering meals, providing comfort items, or simply spending time chatting with patients who may be feeling lonely.

- **Senior Services -** Help seniors in your community by volunteering with organizations that provide services such as transportation to medical appointments or grocery shopping assistance. You can also visit seniors who may be homebound and provide companionship.
- **Political Campaigns -** Get involved in local politics and campaigns by volunteering for candidates whose values align with yours. You can canvas neighborhoods, make phone calls, or even help organize events to support the campaign's message.
- **Art Therapy -** Help others express themselves through art by volunteering with organizations that offer art therapy programs for those with physical or mental disabilities. You don't need to be an artist yourself; just a willingness to help others explore their creativity.
- **Crisis Hotline -** Provide emotional support and guidance to those in need by volunteering with crisis hotlines like the National Suicide Prevention Lifeline or the Crisis Text Line. Training is provided, and you can make a difference from the comfort of your own home.
- **Community Gardening -** Get your hands dirty and help beautify your community by volunteering at a local community garden. You'll get some exercise, fresh air, and the satisfaction of knowing you're contributing to a greener world.

- **Youth Sports Coaching -** Share your love of sports by coaching youth teams in your area. Not only will you help kids develop skills on the field or court, but you'll also serve as a positive role model and mentor.
- **Fundraising Events -** Use your organizational skills to plan and execute fundraising events for local charities or non-profits. From bake sales to silent auctions, there are endless opportunities to raise money for causes you care about.

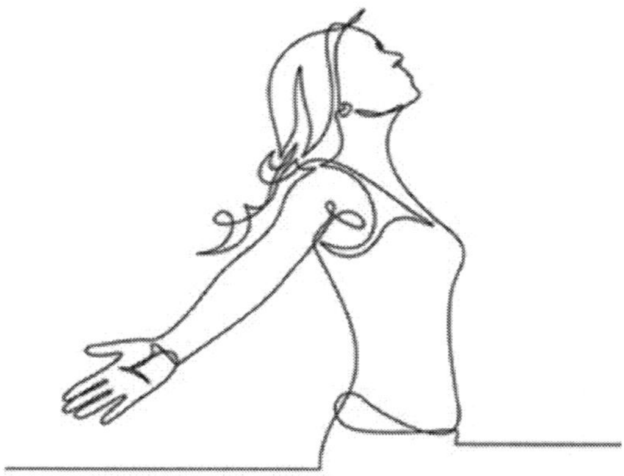

Passing on Your Wisdom: The Joys and Benefits of Mentoring

Remember the wealth of knowledge and experience you've gained over the years. Mentoring others is not only a way to give back to your community, but also a fulfi lling way to stay engaged and active in retirement. In this chapter, we will explore various ways to share your expertise with others and make a positive impact on their lives.

- **Teach a Skill -** Do you have a talent or skill that you've honed over the years? Why not share it with someone who's interested in learning? Whether it's baking, woodworking, or playing an instrument, there's likely someone out there who would love to learn from you. Reach out to local community centers or schools to see if they have any classes or programs where you could offer your expertise.
- **Mentor a Young Professional -** Many young people are just starting out in their careers and could benefit from the guidance of someone who has been there before. Consider volunteering as a mentor through organizations like SCORE or your local Chamber of Commerce. You could help someone navigate the ins and outs of their industry, provide feedback on their work, and offer advice for career growth.
- **Volunteer at a Retirement Community -** Retirement communities are often looking for volunteers to lead activities or simply spend time with residents. Consider offering your time as a mentor figure for those who may be feeling lonely or isolated. Share stories about your own experiences and listen to theirs in return.
- **Start a Book Club -** Love reading? Start a book club where members can discuss books that relate to their professional fields or interests. Use this as an opportunity to share your own insights and perspectives based on your life experiences.
- **Lead Workshops -** Consider leading workshops on topics related to your profession or hobbies at local libraries, community centers, or even online platforms like Zoom! This is an ex-

cellent way to pass along valuable skills while also connecting with others in meaningful ways.

- **Offer to be a Mentor at a Local College -** Many colleges and universities have mentorship programs that connect students with experienced professionals in their desired fields. Reach out to your local college or university to see if they have any opportunities available.

- **Volunteer as a Coach -** Do you have experience playing sports? Consider volunteering as a coach for local youth teams or community leagues. You could help young athletes develop their skills and build confidence, all while sharing your love of the game.

- **Host a Workshop on Financial Planning -** Retirement often involves managing finances more carefully than during our working years. Share your knowledge by hosting workshops on financial planning, budgeting, and investing at local community centers or libraries.

- **Start a Business Incubator -** Have you always been an entrepreneur at heart? Consider starting a business incubator where you can mentor young entrepreneurs and share your own experiences building successful businesses.

- **Join an Online Mentoring Platform -** There are many online platforms like MentorMe that connect mentors with mentees from around the world. Consider joining one of these platforms to share your expertise and connect with people from diverse backgrounds who may benefit from your guidance

- **Offer to be a Language Exchange Partner -** Do you speak another language fluently? Consider offering your skills as a language exchange partner for someone who is trying to learn that language. This can be done in person or virtually through platforms like Skype or Zoom.
- **Host a Cooking Workshop -** If you love cooking, consider hosting a workshop where you can share your favorite recipes and techniques with others. This is an excellent opportunity to bond with others over food while also passing along valuable culinary skills.
- **Volunteer at a Career Center -** Many career centers offer free workshops and counseling sessions for job seekers. Consider volunteering your time to help others write resumes, prepare for interviews, and develop their professional networks.
- **Become a Big Brother/Sister -** Organizations like Big Brothers Big Sisters connect adult mentors with young people who could benefit from positive role models in their lives. Consider becoming a mentor to a child or adolescent in need of support and guidance.
- **Start a Podcast -** Podcasts are an increasingly popular way to share knowledge and experiences with others around the world. Consider starting your own podcast on topics related to your profession or interests as a way of passing along your expertise while also building connections with listeners.

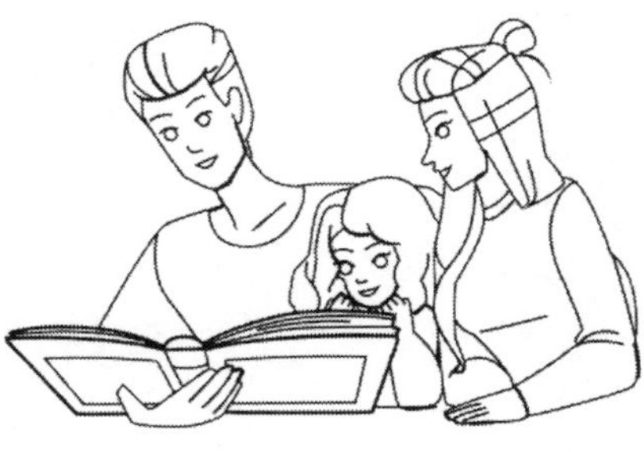

Embrace Community by Joining or Starting a Club

It's important to keep yourself engaged and active. One great way to do so is by joining a club or starting one of your own. In this chapter, we'll explore the benefits of being part of a community with shared interests and provide ideas for clubs that will keep you socializing and learning in retirement.

- **Wine Tasting Club -** Gather with fellow wine enthusiasts to sample different wines from around the world. Each member can bring their favorite bottle to share, and you can learn about tasting techniques, food pairings, and the history of winemaking.

- **Nature Photography Club -** Explore the great outdoors while improving your photography skills. Members can plan outings to local parks or nature reserves, where you can capture stunning images of wildlife, landscapes, and more. Share your photos with the group for feedback and inspiration.

- **Creative Writing Club -** Unleash your inner author by joining a creative writing club. Whether you're a seasoned writer or just starting out, this club provides a supportive environment to share your work and receive constructive feedback from other members.

- **Cooking Club -** If you enjoy trying out new recipes and experimenting in the kitchen, consider joining a cooking club. Each meeting can have a different theme or cuisine, allowing members to expand their culinary horizons while enjoying delicious meals together.

- **Travel Club -** Plan exciting trips with fellow adventurers who share your passion for exploring new destinations. Choose destinations that interest the group, whether it's visiting historical landmarks in Europe or hiking through national parks in North America.
- **Book Club -** Join a book club to discuss and analyze your favorite reads with other book lovers. You can choose a different book each month or focus on a specific genre, author, or theme.
- **Language Exchange Club -** Learn a new language or practice one you already know by joining a language exchange club. Members can take turns teaching and practicing different languages, providing an opportunity to learn from native speakers and improve your conversational skills.
- **Board Game Club -** Spend your afternoons playing classic board games like Monopoly, Scrabble, or Chess with other retirees who enjoy friendly competition. This is also an excellent way to exercise your mind while having fun.
- **Gardening Club -** If you have a green thumb or want to learn more about gardening, join a gardening club where members share tips on growing plants, flowers, and vegetables in their backyards or community gardens.
- **Volunteer Club -** Give back to the community by joining a volunteer club that supports local charities or non-profit organizations in need of assistance. You'll not only make new friends but also feel fulfilled by helping others in meaningful ways.

- **Dance Club -** Join a dance club to learn new moves and socialize with other retirees who enjoy dancing. You can learn different styles of dance, such as ballroom, salsa, or swing.
- **Film Club -** If you're a movie buff, join a film club where members watch and discuss movies together. You can choose a different genre or theme each month and share your thoughts on the films you watch.
- **Fitness Club -** Stay active and healthy by joining a fitness club that offers group exercise classes like yoga, Pilates, or Zumba. This is also an excellent way to meet other retirees who prioritize their health and wellness.
- **Music Club -** Join a music club to listen to and discuss different genres of music with other retirees who appreciate good tunes. You can even start a band or sing in a choir together!
- **Tech Club -** Learn about the latest technology trends and gadgets by joining a tech club that focuses on exploring new digital tools and software programs. This is also an excellent opportunity to improve your computer skills.

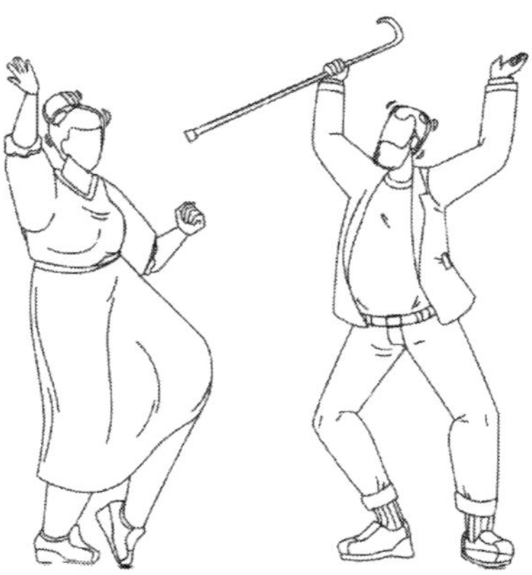

Making a Difference: Get Involved in Politics

Politics can be an exciting and fulfilling way to stay engaged with the world around you during your retirement years. Whether it's volunteering for a political campaign, attending town hall meetings, or even running for local office yourself, there are plenty of ways to become involved in the democratic process. In this chapter, we'll explore some of the best ways to get involved in politics and make a difference in your community.

- **Attend a city council meeting -** Spend an evening listening to local politicians discuss issues that affect your community. You may be surprised at how engaging and informative these meetings can be.

- **Volunteer for a political campaign -** Whether it's for a local school board or state representative, volunteering for a political campaign is a great way to meet new people and learn about the political process.

- **Participate in a protest -** If there's an issue you're passionate about, consider joining a protest or rally to show your support. Retirement gives you the freedom to speak out on issues that matter to you.

- **Start your own grassroots movement -** If you can't find an organization that aligns with your values, consider starting your own! Gather like-minded individuals and work together towards making change in your community.

- **Run for office -** Retirement is the perfect time to run for office! Consider running for city council or even mayor if you're feeling ambitious. Your life experience and passion can make all the difference in improving your community.

- **Join a local political club -** Check out any local political clubs or organizations that align with your beliefs and values. This is a great way to meet like-minded individuals and stay informed about political issues.

- **Attend a town hall meeting -** Attend a town hall meeting hosted by an elected official to hear their thoughts on current events and ask them questions directly.

- **Work at the polls -** Consider working as a poll worker during elections. You'll gain an inside look at the voting process and help ensure fair elections.

- **Lobby for a cause you believe in -** If there's an issue you're passionate about, consider lobbying your elected officials to make change happen.

- **Get involved with voter registration efforts -** Help register new voters by volunteering with organizations that work towards increasing voter turnout in your community.

- **Attend a political fundraiser -** Attend a political fundraiser and learn about the candidates running for office. This is a great way to meet new people and support causes that align with your values.

- **Write letters to elected officials -** Write letters to your elected officials advocating for issues you care about. This can have a big impact on policy decisions.

- **Join a local advocacy group -** Join an advocacy group focused on issues you care about, such as environmental protection or social justice.
- **Participate in a mock trial -** Consider participating in a mock trial at your local courthouse, where you can learn about the legal system and how it affects politics.
- **Teach civics classes -** Share your knowledge of politics by teaching civics classes at local schools or community centers. This is a great way to inspire future generations to get involved in politics and make a difference in their communities.

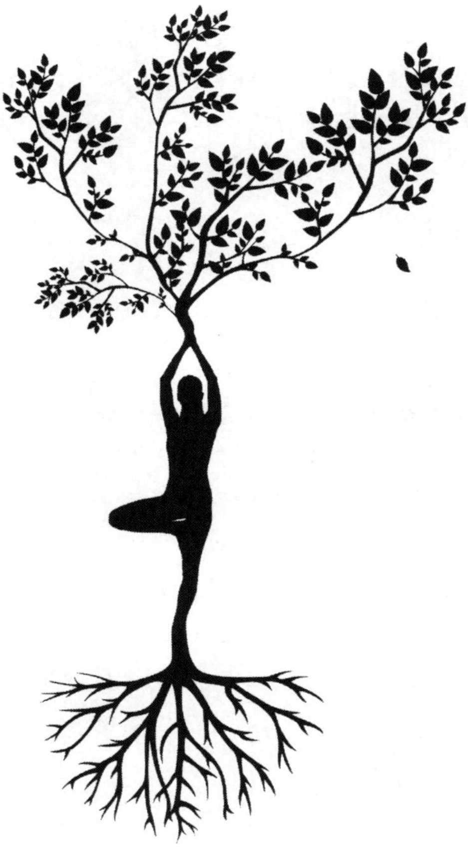

The Power of Charitable Giving

Being charitable not only helps those in need, but it also brings a sense of fulfillment and purpose to our own lives. In this chapter, we'll explore various ways to make a positive impact on our communities and beyond. From volunteering at local organizations to organizing donation drives, these activities will leave a lasting impression on both ourselves and those we help.

- **Random Acts of Kindness -** Make a list of small but meaningful things you can do for strangers throughout the day, such as buying someone's coffee or leaving a note of encouragement on a car windshield.
- **Volunteer Vacation -** Plan a trip with purpose by signing up for a volunteer vacation. Whether it's building homes in a foreign country or working at an animal sanctuary, you'll make a difference while exploring new places.
- **Donate Your Skills -** Consider donating your expertise to a non-profit organization that could benefit from your knowledge. For example, if you're an accountant, offer to help with their financial statements.
- **Host a Charity Event -** Use your retirement as an opportunity to give back by hosting a charity event. It could be anything from a bake sale to a silent auction, and all proceeds will go towards helping those in need.
- **Give Back Locally -** Research local charities and organizations in your community that could use some extra support. Whether it's volunteering at the local food bank or donating clothes to the homeless shelter, there are plenty of ways to make a difference close to home.

- **Organize a Fundraiser -** Put your event planning skills to good use by organizing a fundraiser for a cause you care about. From charity walks to benefit concerts, there are many creative ways to raise money and awareness.
- **Donate Blood -** Consider donating blood or platelets to help save lives. Many hospitals and blood banks offer donation opportunities, and the process is relatively quick and easy.
- **Environmental Stewardship -** Take care of the planet by participating in environmental stewardship activities such as cleaning up litter in your community or volunteering at a local nature center.
- **Pay it Forward -** Challenge yourself to pay it forward each day by doing something kind for others without expecting anything in return. It could be as simple as holding the door open for someone or giving a compliment to a stranger on the street.
- **Participate in a Charity Walk or Run -** Sign up for a charity walk or run to raise money and awareness for a cause you care about. It's a great way to get active and make a positive impact.
- **Host a Donation Drive -** Organize a donation drive for items such as clothing, books, or household goods to benefit those in need. You can partner with local organizations to distribute the donations.
- **Meals on Wheels -** Volunteer with Meals on Wheels to deliver meals to homebound seniors in your community. It's a great way to provide companionship and ensure that seniors have access to nutritious food.

- **Support Small Businesses -** Consider supporting small businesses owned by underrepresented groups by shopping at their stores or purchasing their products online.
- **Create Care Packages -** Assemble care packages for those experiencing homelessness or other difficult situations. Include items such as toiletries, socks, and snacks, along with notes of encouragement.

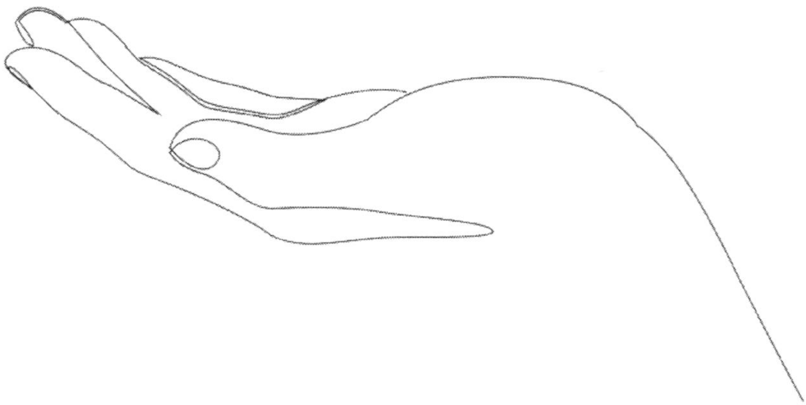

ACHIEVING PERSONAL GROWTH AND FULFILLMENT

Retirement is the perfect time to focus on personal growth and self-improvement. After years of working and raising a family, it's finally your time to explore new interests, learn new skills, and discover more about yourself. In this chapter, we'll explore a variety of activities that will help you expand your horizons, challenge yourself, and reach new heights in your personal development journey. Whether you want to learn a new language, take up painting, or start writing a memoir, there's no better time than now to invest in yourself and create the life you've always dreamed of. So let's dive in and get started on this exciting new chapter in your life!

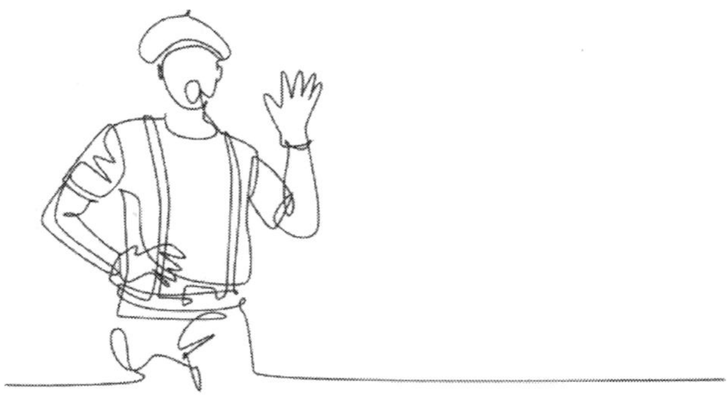

Crafting a Meaningful Retirement Experience: Creating Your Ultimate Bucket List

This chapter is dedicated to helping you build a bucket list that will inspire and excite you. From adrenaline-pumping adventures to creative pursuits, there's something for everyone. So grab a pen and paper, and let's get started on creating experiences that will stay with you forever.

- **Write Your Memoir -** You've lived an interesting life and now is the time to share your story with others. Writing your memoir can be a fun and fulfilling experience that allows you to reflect on your past and leave behind something for future generations.

- **Take Up Photography -** With all the free time retirement brings, why not explore your creative side? Photography is a great way to capture memories and express yourself artistically. Invest in a good camera and take classes or watch tutorials online.
- **Go on a Road Trip -** There's nothing quite like hitting the open road and exploring new places at your own pace. Plan out a route, pack up the car, and set off on an adventure with no real destination in mind. It's all about enjoying the journey!
- **Learn an Instrument -** Always wanted to play the guitar or piano? Retirement is a great time to pick up a new hobby and learn how to play an instrument. Take lessons or use online resources like YouTube tutorials.
- **Attend a TED Talk -** TED Talks are informative and inspiring lectures given by experts in various fields. Many cities host local TED events, making it easy for you to attend in person and learn something new.
- **Build Something -** Whether it's woodworking, pottery, or knitting, building something with your own hands can be incredibly rewarding. Join a class or workshop to learn new skills and create something you can be proud of.
- **Take a Cooking Class -** Always wanted to learn how to cook Italian cuisine or bake the perfect croissant? Retirement is the perfect time to take a cooking class and develop new culinary skills.

- **Learn a New Sport -** Retirement doesn't have to mean slowing down. Learn a new sport like golf, tennis, or pickleball and stay active while also having fun.
- **Start a Garden -** Gardening is a great way to get outside and connect with nature. Whether you have a small balcony or a large backyard, starting a garden can be both therapeutic and rewarding.
- **Take an Art Class -** Painting, drawing, sculpting – there are endless possibilities when it comes to art classes. Find one that interests you and let your creativity flow.
- **Attend a Music Festival -** Music festivals are not just for young people! There are many festivals that cater to all ages and musical tastes. Pack up your tent and enjoy live music in the great outdoors.

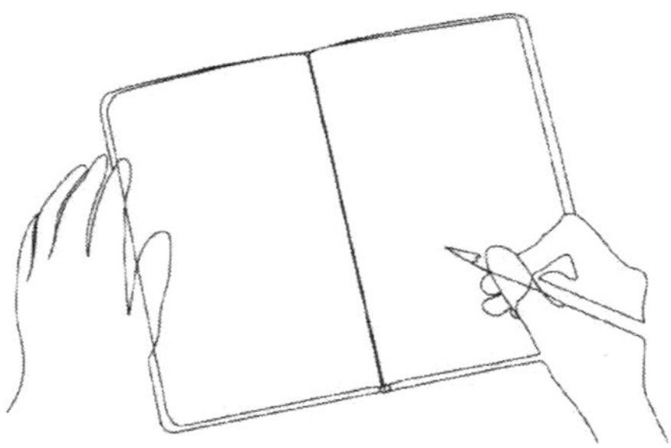

Cultivating Meaningful Connections and Strengthening Bonds

From simple yet meaningful gestures to exciting adventures, these activities aim to deepen bonds and create lasting memories. Whether it's spending quality time with grandchildren or embarking on a romantic getaway, there's something for everyone in this section.

- **Host a Game Night -** Gather your friends and family for a fun night of games. From classic board games to party games, there are plenty of options to choose from. Make it even more special by creating custom game boards or prizes.
- **Plan a Group Trip -** Traveling with loved ones can be an unforgettable experience. Plan a group trip with friends or family members and explore new destinations together. Whether it's a road trip across the country or an international adventure, traveling as a group can bring you closer together.
- **Create a Memory Book -** Collect photos and mementos from special moments in your relationships and compile them into a memory book. This activity not only allows you to reminisce on past experiences but also creates something tangible that you can share with loved ones for years to come.
- **Attend a Cultural Event -** Discover new cultures and experiences by attending cultural events with your loved ones. Look for local festivals, concerts, or exhibitions that showcase different traditions and art forms. You'll not only deepen your relationships but also expand your horizons.
- **Volunteer Together -** Spend time with your loved ones while giving back to the community. Look for volunteer opportunities that align with your shared interests or passions. Whether it's serving meals at a shelter, cleaning up a park, or reading to children, volunteering can strengthen bonds and create meaningful memories.
- **Have a Picnic -** Enjoy the outdoors while spending quality time with loved ones by having a picnic. Choose a scenic location,

pack some delicious food, and bring along games or activities for added fun.

- **Take a Dance Class -** Learning to dance together can be a fun and romantic activity that strengthens bonds. Sign up for a dance class with your partner or friend and try out different styles like salsa, ballroom, or swing.

- **Create Art Together -** Explore your creative sides by making art together with loved ones. Whether it's painting, drawing, or sculpting, creating something together can be an enriching experience that brings you closer together. Display your artwork in your home as a reminder of the special moments you shared while making it.

- **Host a Potluck -** Bring your loved ones together for a delicious meal by hosting a potluck. Each person can bring their favorite dish to share, creating a diverse and tasty spread. Make it even more fun by setting up a theme or challenge, like making dishes from different countries.

- **Play Sports Together -** Get active with your friends or family members by playing sports together. Choose a sport that everyone enjoys, like basketball, soccer, or tennis, and spend time bonding while getting some exercise.

- **Write Letters to Each Other -** In this digital age, taking the time to write a heartfelt letter can be a meaningful way to deepen relationships. Write letters to loved ones expressing your feelings and gratitude for them, and encourage them to do the same.

- **Take a Photography Class -** Capture memories together by taking a photography class with your loved ones. Learn new techniques and skills while exploring interesting locations in your community or beyond. You'll not only deepen your relationships but also have beautiful photos as keepsakes of your experiences together.

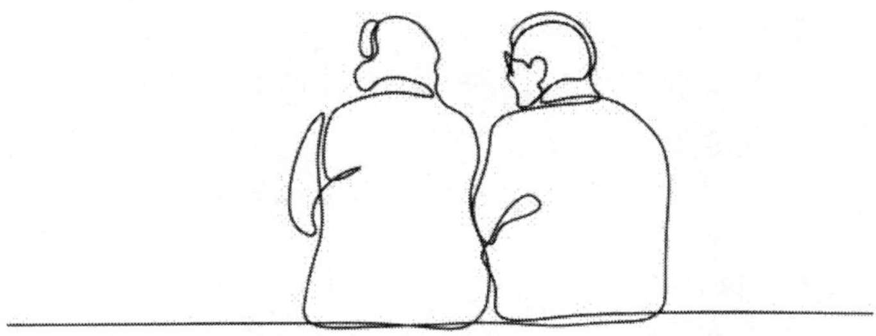

Entrepreneurship in Retirement: Turning Your Passion into a Profitable Venture

Starting a business can be an excellent way to stay engaged and productive while also generating income. Whether you have a passion project or a unique skill set to offer, we'll provide tips and resources to help you turn your ideas into a successful venture.

- **Pet Pampering -** If you love animals, why not start a business that caters to pets? From dog walking to grooming, there are plenty of opportunities in this field. Consider offering specialized services like pet massage or even pet acupuncture.

- **Meal Delivery -** Many retirees are looking for healthy and convenient meal options. Starting a meal delivery service can be a great way to fill this need. Focus on fresh, organic ingredients and offer customizable menus to appeal to a variety of tastes.

- **Senior Fitness Classes -** As more people enter retirement age, the demand for fitness classes tailored specifically for seniors is growing. Offer low-impact exercises like yoga or tai chi, or try something new like water aerobics.

- **Home Organization -** Downsizing can be overwhelming for many retirees. Offer your services as a home organizer to help them declutter and simplify their living spaces.

- **Online Tutoring -** With the rise of online learning, starting an online tutoring business can be a lucrative venture. Focus on subjects you're passionate about and set your own schedule for maximum flexibility.

- **Personal Concierge -** Many retirees want to enjoy their newfound free time and may need help running errands or planning events. Offer personalized concierge services like grocery shopping, scheduling appointments, and even travel planning.
- **Mobile Car Detailing -** If you love cars, consider starting a mobile car detailing business. Travel to clients' homes or offices and offer specialized services like waxing and interior cleaning.
- **Customized Gift Baskets -** Starting a gift basket business can be a fun way to showcase your creativity while helping others celebrate special occasions. Focus on customized baskets tailored to each recipient's interests or hobbies.
- **Home Staging -** As the real estate market continues to boom, home staging has become increasingly popular. Help homeowners prepare their homes for sale by offering home staging services that showcase the property's best features.
- **Antique Appraisal -** If you have an eye for antiques, consider starting an antique appraisal business. Offer your expertise to collectors looking to buy or sell valuable items, or host antique appraisal events at local fairs and markets.
- **Social Media Management -** With the rise of social media, many businesses are looking for help managing their online presence. Offer social media management services to small businesses or individuals looking to build their personal brand.
- **Event Planning -** If you love planning parties and events, consider starting an event planning business. From weddings to corporate events, there is always demand for someone who can handle the logistics and details of an event.

- **Personal Shopping -** Many busy professionals don't have time to shop for themselves or need help finding the perfect outfit for a special occasion. Offer personal shopping services and use your fashion expertise to help clients look and feel their best.

- **Freelance Writing or Editing -** If you have a way with words, consider offering freelance writing or editing services. Write blog posts or articles on topics you're passionate about, or help others polish their own writing projects.

Staying Active in Retirement

Stay physically active and maintain a healthy lifestyle. This chapter will explore various activities that will keep you moving and help you discover new ways to enjoy exercise. From hiking scenic trails to trying out dance classes, there's something for everyone to enjoy and stay fit during retirement.

- **Aqua Zumba -** Who says exercise can't be fun? Aqua Zumba brings the party to the pool, combining dance moves with water resistance for a low-impact workout that's easy on joints. Plus, there's no better way to beat the heat than by cooling off in the water.

- **Pickleball -** Looking for a new sport to try? Pickleball may just be your new favorite game! It's a cross between tennis, badminton, and ping pong, played on a smaller court with paddles and a wiffle ball. It's easy to learn but challenging enough to keep you coming back for more.

- **Tai Chi -** If you're looking for something more calming, give Tai Chi a try! This ancient Chinese practice focuses on slow movements combined with deep breathing techniques, promoting relaxation and stress relief while also improving balance and flexibility.

- **Hiking with Llamas -** Want to add some furry friends to your outdoor adventures? Consider hiking with llamas! These gentle creatures can carry your gear while you explore scenic trails together. It's a unique experience that combines physical activity with animal companionship.

- **Trampoline Fitness -** Who says trampolines are just for kids? Trampoline fitness classes are a fun way to get your heart rate up while bouncing on a mini-trampoline. The low-impact workout is easy on joints but still provides a full-body workout.

- **Urban Poling -** Walking with poles may seem like something only Nordic skiers do, but urban poling is becoming increasingly popular as a form of exercise. Using special poles designed for walking, this activity engages more muscles than regular walking and can improve posture and balance.

- **Slacklining -** If you have good balance and want to challenge yourself even further, give slacklining a try! This activity involves balancing on a flat nylon webbing stretched between two anchor points. It's great for improving core strength, balance, and focus. Plus, it's always impressive to show off at social gatherings!

- **Barre Fitness -** Looking for a low-impact workout that combines ballet-inspired moves with strength training? Give barre fitness a try! This popular exercise routine uses a ballet barre as support while you perform small, isolated movements that target specific muscle groups.
- **Disc Golf -** If you enjoy outdoor activities and want to try something new, disc golf might be right up your alley. Similar to traditional golf, disc golf involves throwing specially-designed discs at targets on a course. It's a great way to get some fresh air and exercise while enjoying the company of friends.
- **Hoop Dancing -** Remember hula hooping from your childhood? Hoop dancing takes it to the next level by combining dance moves with spinning hoops around your body. It's a fun way to improve coordination, flexibility, and core strength.
- **Belly Dancing -** Want to try something exotic and sensual? Consider belly dancing! This Middle Eastern dance style involves fluid movements of the hips and torso, providing a full-body workout that can also boost confidence and self-expression.
- **Acro Yoga -** Looking for an activity that combines elements of yoga, acrobatics, and Thai massage? Give Acro Yoga a try! This partner practice involves one person acting as the "base" while another person performs yoga poses on top of them. It's a great way to build trust, communication skills, and physical strength together with a friend or partner.

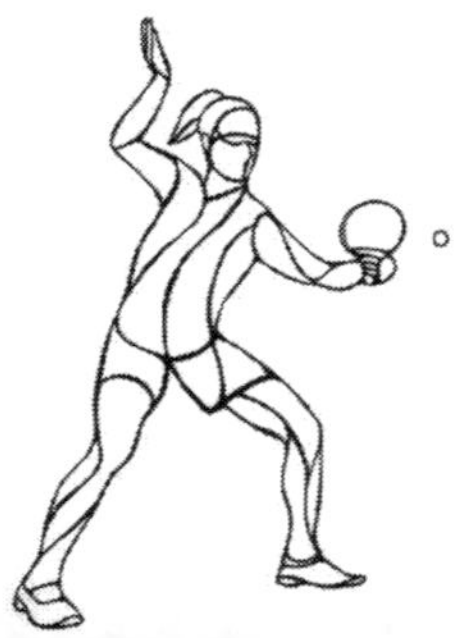

Discover the Joy of Writing and Possibly Profit from it

Writing can be a fulfilling activity that provides an outlet for creativity and self-expression. Whether it's penning a memoir or trying your hand at fiction, writ-ing is an excellent way to keep the mind sharp and engaged. In this chapter, we'll explore various writing activities that will not only provide enjoyment but also have the potential to generate income.

- **Write your memoirs** - Everyone has a story to tell, and retirement provides the perfect opportunity to finally write it down. Share your life experiences with others by writing your memoirs. Not only will it serve as a keepsake for you and your family, but it could also potentially be published for profit.
- **Start a blog** - Blogging is an excellent way to share your thoughts and opinions on various topics with the world. It's easy to get started with platforms like WordPress or Blogger, and there are countless tutorials available online to help you along the way.
- **Write greeting cards** - If you have a talent for creative writing, consider channeling that skill into creating greeting cards. There's always a demand for unique and heartfelt cards, especially during holidays and special occasions.
- **Become a freelance writer** - Retirement doesn't have to mean the end of your career. If you enjoy writing, consider becoming a freelance writer. There are countless websites where you can find work as a freelance writer, such as Upwork or Fiverr.
- **Participate in writing contests** - Many publications hold regular writing contests throughout the year, offering cash prizes

for winning entries. Participating in these contests can not only help improve your skills as a writer but also give you an opportunity to win some extra cash.

- **Write a cookbook** - If you're passionate about cooking and have some favorite recipes, consider compiling them into a cookbook. You could even include personal anecdotes or stories to make it more engaging.
- **Pen pal program** - Participate in a pen pal program to connect with people from all over the world through handwritten letters. It's a great way to practice your writing skills while also making new friends.
- **Write fan fiction** - If you're a fan of a particular book, movie or TV series, consider writing fan fiction based on the characters and storyline. It can be a fun and creative way to explore your imagination.
- **Create an e-book** - With self-publishing platforms like Kindle Direct Publishing or Smashwords, it's easy to create and publish an e-book. Write about any topic that interests you and share it with the world.
- **Start a journaling group** - Join or start a journaling group where members can share their daily reflections and experiences with each other. It's an excellent way to stay motivated and accountable for your writing goals while also building connections with others who share similar interests.
- **Write a travel guide** - If you love to travel, consider writing a travel guide based on your experiences. Share tips and recommendations for places to visit, eat and stay with other travelers.

- **Create a family history book** - Research your family tree and document your findings in a book format. Share it with your family members so they can learn more about their roots.
- **Write poetry** - Explore your creative side by writing poetry. It's an excellent way to express emotions and thoughts in a unique and artistic way.
- **Start a memoir writing group** - Join or start a memoir writing group where members can share their life stories with each other. It's an excellent way to get feedback on your writing and connect with others who have similar experiences.
- **Write short stories** - Challenge yourself by writing short stories with specific themes or prompts. It's an excellent way to improve your storytelling skills while also having fun with the creative process.

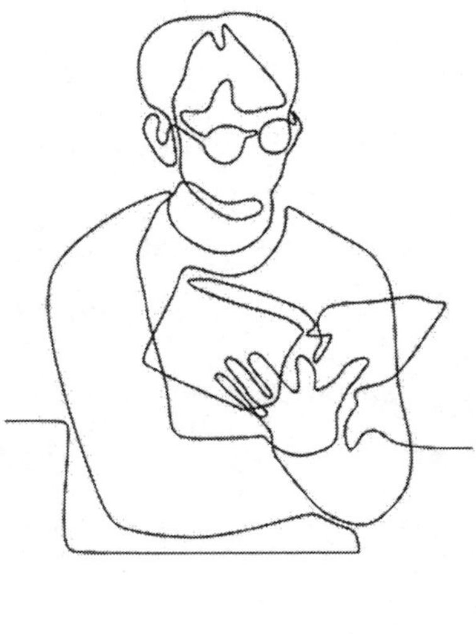

Challenging Yourself Mentally

Keep your mind active and challenged. In this chapter, we'll explore activities that will exercise your brain and keep you mentally sharp. From stimulating games to learning new skills, these challenges will not only keep you entertained but also help you maintain cognitive function as you age. So let's dive into some exciting ways to challenge yourself mentally during your retirement years.

- **Sudoku Challenges -** Give your brain a workout with Sudoku puzzles. These number-based logic games range in difficulty from easy to expert level, so you'll always have a challenge ahead of you. You can find Sudoku books at local bookstores or try online versions for free.

- **Memory Games -** Challenge yourself with memory games like Simon Says, Concentration, or Memory Match. These games help improve cognitive function and memory retention while providing hours of fun.

- **Mindful Meditation -** Engage in mindful meditation practices to reduce stress and improve focus and concentration. Apps like Headspace, Calm, or Insight Timer offer guided meditations and mindfulness exercises that are perfect for beginners.

- **Chess or Strategy Games -** Play games like chess, checkers, or other strategy games to exercise your mind and improve critical thinking skills. Join local clubs or play online with friends to keep the challenge fresh.

- **Crossword Puzzles -** Work on crossword puzzles to keep your vocabulary sharp and improve problem-solving skills. Challenge yourself with difficult puzzles or compete with friends to see who can finish first.

- **Read Challenging Books -** Read books that challenge you intellectually and expand your knowledge in new areas. Try reading classic literature, non-fiction books about science or history, or books on philosophy to stretch your mental muscles.

- **Attend Lectures or Conferences -** Attend lectures or conferences on topics that interest you to learn new things and engage in discussions with experts in the field. Local universities often offer free lectures on various subjects that are open to the public.

- **Online Courses -** Take online courses on topics that interest you to learn new skills and expand your knowledge. Websites like Coursera or Udemy offer a wide range of courses on various subjects, from computer science to creative writing.

- **Brain Teasers -** Solve brain teasers like riddles, logic puzzles, or math problems to keep your mind sharp and improve problem-solving skills. You can find these types of puzzles in books or online.

- **Attend Trivia Nights -** Attend trivia nights at local bars or restaurants to challenge yourself with random facts and compete with friends. Trivia games help improve memory retention and recall while providing social interaction.

- **Play Strategy Video Games -** Play strategy video games like Civilization or Age of Empires to exercise your mind and improve critical thinking skills. These games require planning, decision-making, and resource management, all of which are great for keeping the mind active.

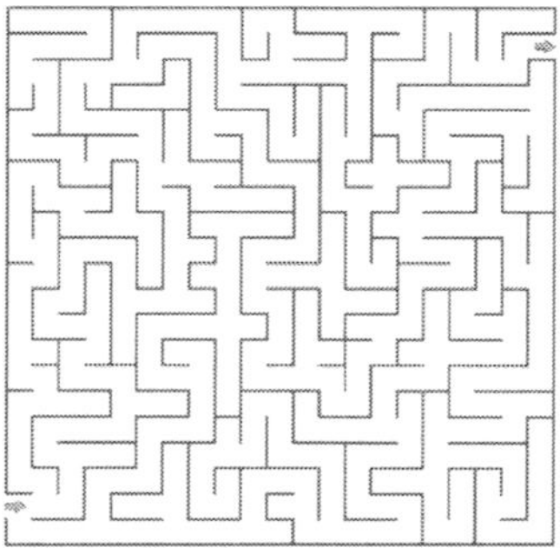

Challenging Yourself Physically

Stay active and healthy. In this chapter, we'll explore exciting physical challenges that will push your limits and help you maintain a strong body and mind. From adrenaline-fueled adventures to endurance-building activities, you'll discover new ways to challenge yourself and enjoy all that life has to off er.

- **Stand Up Paddleboarding -** If you're looking for a fun and challenging way to stay active, try stand up paddleboarding (SUP). This water sport not only provides a full-body workout but also helps improve your balance and core strength. Plus, it's a great way to enjoy the outdoors and soak up some vitamin D.

- **Indoor Rock Climbing -** If you're not quite ready to conquer the great outdoors, try indoor rock climbing. This activity challenges both your physical and mental abilities as you navigate different routes and heights. It's a great workout for your arms, legs, and core, while also improving your problem-solving skills.

- **Aerial Yoga -** Take your yoga practice to new heights with aerial yoga. Using a hammock suspended from the ceiling, this form of yoga allows you to perform poses in mid-air, providing a unique challenge for your body and mind. It also helps improve flexibility, balance, and upper body strength.

- **Parkour -** For those who like a bit of adrenaline with their workouts, parkour is an excellent option. This urban sport involves using your body to navigate obstacles such as walls, railings, and stairs in a fluid motion. It requires strength, agility, and quick thinking but can be incredibly rewarding once you master it.

- **Martial Arts -** Whether it's karate or taekwondo or any other discipline that interests you; martial arts is an excellent way to challenge yourself physically while also learning self-defense techniques. It requires discipline and focus while improving flexibility, strength, speed & coordination skills which will keep you fit even in retirement age!

- **Dance Fitness -** Spice up your exercise routine with dance fitness classes such as Zumba, salsa, or hip hop. These high-energy workouts are not only a great way to stay active but also help improve coordination and balance while having fun.

- **Surfing -** If you live near the coast, surfing is an excellent way to challenge yourself physically and mentally. It requires strength, balance, and endurance as you navigate the waves on a board. Plus, it's a fantastic way to enjoy the ocean and soak up some sun.

- **CrossFit -** For those who like a bit of competition with their workouts, CrossFit may be the perfect fit. This high-intensity workout program combines elements of weightlifting, gymnastics, and cardio to provide a total-body workout that challenges both your physical and mental abilities.
- **Kayaking -** Another water sport that's great for staying active is kayaking. It provides a full-body workout as you paddle through calm lakes or choppy rivers while enjoying the scenery around you.
- **Pole Fitness -** Pole fitness is a fun and challenging way to stay active while building strength and flexibility. This form of exercise involves performing acrobatic moves on a vertical pole, which requires upper body and core strength, as well as balance and coordination.
- **Tai Chi -** Tai chi is a low-impact martial art that focuses on slow, flowing movements and deep breathing. It's an excellent way to improve balance, flexibility, and relaxation while also being gentle on the joints.
- **Rowing -** If you're looking for a full-body workout that's easy on the joints, try rowing. This low-impact exercise provides an excellent cardiovascular workout while also toning your arms, legs, back, and core.
- **Trail Running -** Take your running off-road by hitting the trails! Trail running provides a fantastic cardio workout while also challenging your balance and coordination as you navigate uneven terrain.

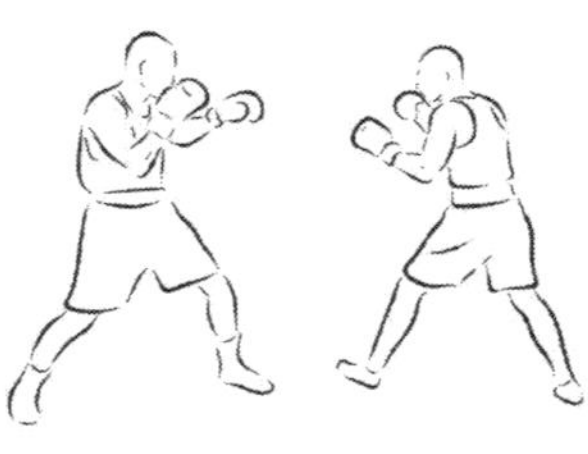

HAVING FUN

Retirement is a time for relaxation, rejuvenation and most importantly, having fun! After years of hard work and dedication to your career, it's finally time to indulge in activities that bring you joy and make your heart happy. This chapter is dedicated to helping you discover unique and enjoyable ways to spend your newfound freedom. From exploring new hobbies to traveling the world, we've got you covered. So sit back, relax and get ready to have some fun!

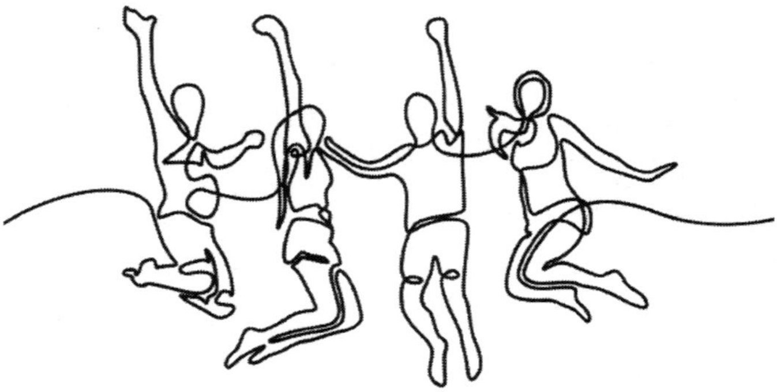

Creating Unforgettable Memories by Enjoying Events That Interest You

Continue pursu-ing your passions and interests. In this chapter, we explore various events that will allow you to do just that. From cultural festivals to sporting events, there's something for everyone. Get ready to immerse yourself in new experiences and create unforgettable memories.

- **Art Crawl -** Spend an afternoon exploring different art galleries in your city or town. Many galleries offer free admission, and you may even have the opportunity to meet local artists and learn about their work.

- **Volunteer at a Music Festival -** Music festivals are always in need of volunteers to help with tasks like ticket sales, parking, and crowd control. In exchange for your time, you'll get free admission to the festival and the chance to see some amazing performances.
- **Attend a Film Screening -** Check out local film societies or independent theaters in your area for screenings of classic films or new independent movies. Many venues offer discounted tickets for seniors, so you can enjoy a movie without breaking the bank.
- **Attend a Poetry Reading -** Check out local poetry events in your area, such as open mic nights or readings at coffee shops or bookstores. Listening to poetry can be a great way to relax and find inspiration.
- **Visit a Historical Site -** Take a day trip to visit a historical site or museum that interests you. Many museums offer guided tours, which can provide valuable insights into the history and culture of the area.
- **Join a Photography Club -** If you enjoy taking photos, consider joining a photography club in your area. You'll have the opportunity to learn new techniques and share your work with others who appreciate the art form.
- **Participate in Trivia Nights -** Many bars and restaurants host trivia nights, where teams compete for prizes by answering questions on various topics. It's a fun way to exercise your brain

and socialize with friends.

- **Attend a Comedy Show -** Laughter is always good medicine, so why not attend a comedy show? Look for local comedians performing at clubs or theaters near you, or check out touring acts coming through town. You're sure to have a good time!

- **Attend a Local Sports Game -** Whether it's minor league baseball, college football, or high school basketball, attending a local sports game can be a fun way to support your community and connect with other fans.

- **Take a Dance Class -** Always wanted to learn how to salsa or ballroom dance? Retirement is the perfect time to take up dancing as a hobby. Look for classes at community centers or dance studios in your area.

- **Join a Nature Walk Group -** If you enjoy being outdoors and exploring nature, consider joining a nature walk group. You'll have the opportunity to explore local parks and trails while socializing with like-minded individuals.

- **Attend a Wine Tasting -** Many wineries offer tastings where you can sample different wines and learn about the winemaking process. It's a great way to expand your palate and discover new wines that you love.

- **Participate in Community Theater -** Have you ever dreamed of being on stage? Retirement is the perfect time to try out community theater. Many theaters offer auditions for upcoming productions, and even if you don't get cast, there are often opportunities to work behind-the-scenes.

Unforgettable Home Activities

It can be challenging to find ways to make the most of our days. Here are some ideas on how to keep yourself entertained and engaged without leaving the house. From creative projects to relaxing activities, these suggestions will help you make the most of your time at home.

- **DIY Spa Day -** Create your own spa experience at home with a DIY facial, manicure, and pedicure. Use natural ingredients like honey, avocado, and coconut oil for a luxurious pampering session without leaving your house.
- **Virtual Cooking Class -** Sign up for a virtual cooking class with friends or family members. Learn how to make new dishes from around the world while socializing and having fun from the comfort of your own kitchen.
- **Indoor Treasure Hunt -** Create clues and hide treasures around your home for an exciting indoor treasure hunt. This activity is perfect on a rainy day or when you're looking for something fun to do indoors.
- **Movie Marathon -** Plan a movie marathon day with your favorite films or TV shows. Pop some popcorn, grab some snacks, and settle in for a cozy day on the couch.
- **Paint and Sip Night -** Host your own paint and sip night at home with friends or family members. Set up easels, canvas, brushes, and paint supplies and enjoy wine while creating beautiful artwork together.
- **Board Game Tournament -** Host a board game tournament with friends or family members. Choose your favorite games

and play multiple rounds until a winner is declared.

- **DIY Home Decor -** Get crafty and create your own home decor pieces. From painting canvases to making wreaths, there are endless possibilities to add a personal touch to your living space.
- **Virtual Book Club -** Join or start a virtual book club with friends or family members. Discuss books from different genres and authors while enjoying each other's company virtually.
- **Backyard Camping -** Pitch a tent in your backyard, make s'mores over the fire pit, and enjoy the great outdoors without leaving the comfort of your home.
- **Indoor Picnic -** Spread out a blanket on your living room floor and have an indoor picnic with your favorite snacks and beverages. Bonus points for themed decor!
- **DIY Movie Theater -** Transform your living room into a movie theater by setting up a projector, screen, and comfortable seating. Pop some popcorn and enjoy a movie night from the comfort of your own home.
- **Puzzle Challenge -** Choose a challenging puzzle and work on it over several days or weeks with friends or family members. Set up a designated puzzle area in your home for everyone to work on.
- **Virtual Dance Party -** Host a virtual dance party with friends or family members using video conferencing software. Create a playlist of your favorite songs and dance the night away together.

- **Memory Lane Scrapbooking -** Take a trip down memory lane by creating scrapbooks filled with photos, memorabilia, and stories from your past adventures and experiences.

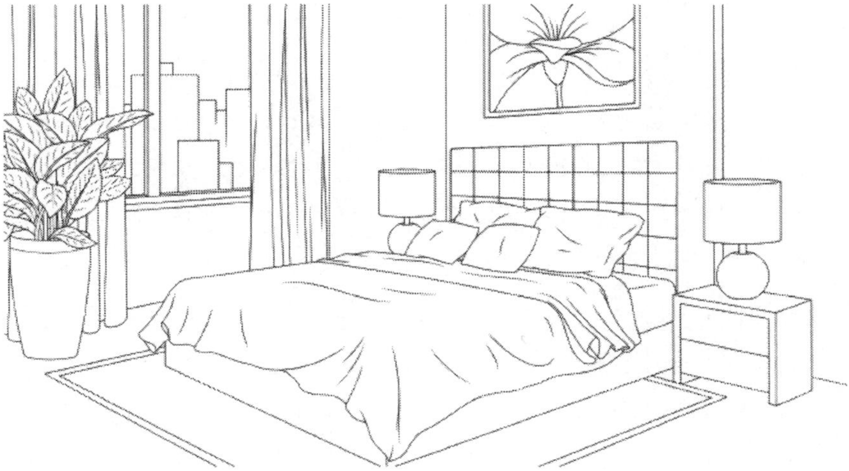

Creating Memorable Culinary Experiences

There is no better way to celebrate than indulging in some of the world's most delicious foodie delights. From savoring exotic flavors to learning new cooking techniques, this chapter will take you on a culinary journey like no other. Get ready to tantalize your taste buds and explore the endless possibilities of gastronomy.

- **Farm-to-Table Tour -** Embark on a farm-to-table tour to learn about locally sourced food and how it's prepared. Meet with farmers, taste fresh produce and indulge in delicious meals made from the ingredients you've just seen harvested. It's a great way to support local businesses and learn more about sustainable farming practices.

- **Cooking Classes -** Take up cooking classes with a professional chef to hone your culinary skills. Learn how to make gourmet dishes, experiment with new flavors, and create your own signature recipes. You'll not only impress your friends and family but also have fun while learning something new.
- **Food Festivals -** Explore food festivals that celebrate different cuisines from around the world. Experience unique flavors, try exotic dishes, and immerse yourself in the culture of each cuisine. From spicy Indian curries to savory Italian pastas, there's something for everyone.
- **Wine Tasting -** Visit local wineries for wine tastings and tours of their vineyards. Learn about the different types of wines, how they're made, and what food pairs well with each one. It's an excellent opportunity to sample some of the best wines in your region while enjoying scenic views.
- **Culinary Road Trip -** Plan a culinary road trip across different regions or countries to explore their unique cuisine. Visit local markets, try street food, dine at Michelin-starred restaurants, and indulge in sweet treats along the way. It's a fun-filled adventure that will leave you with unforgettable memories of delicious food and amazing experiences.
- **Foraging -** Go on a foraging adventure to find wild edible plants and mushrooms. Learn about the different species, how to identify them, and how to prepare them in delicious dishes. It's an eco-friendly way to connect with nature while discovering new flavors.
- **Food Photography -** Take up food photography as a hobby and learn how to capture mouth-watering images of your fa-

vorite dishes. Experiment with different lighting, angles, and props to create stunning visuals that showcase the beauty of food.

- **Molecular Gastronomy -** Attend a molecular gastronomy workshop to explore the science behind cooking and learn how to create innovative dishes using cutting-edge techniques. From foams and gels to liquid nitrogen ice cream, you'll discover a whole new world of culinary possibilities.

- **Homebrewing -** Try your hand at homebrewing beer or making wine from scratch. Learn about the fermentation process, experiment with different ingredients, and create unique blends that reflect your personal taste.

- **Food Swap Parties -** Organize a food swap party with friends where everyone brings their homemade treats to share. From jams and pickles to baked goods and chocolates, it's a fun way to try new foods while bonding over a shared love of cooking and eating delicious treats.

- **Food History Tour -** Take a guided tour of a local museum or historic site that explores the history of food and its impact on culture. Learn about ancient cooking techniques, traditional recipes, and how food has shaped human civilization.

- **Chocolate Making Workshop -** Attend a chocolate making workshop to learn how to create your own decadent chocolates from scratch. Discover the art of tempering chocolate, experiment with different flavors and textures, and take home your own handmade chocolates.

- **Street Food Crawl -** Plan a street food crawl through your city or town to discover hidden gems and hole-in-the-wall eateries that serve up delicious snacks and meals. From tacos and kebabs to dumplings and crepes, there's no shortage of mouth-watering options to try.
- **Cookbook Club -** Join or start a cookbook club where members choose a cookbook each month to cook from together. Share recipes, tips, and stories while enjoying delicious meals made from different cuisines around the world.
- **Pop-Up Restaurant Night -** Host a pop-up restaurant night at home where you invite friends over for an evening of gourmet dining. Create a themed menu, decorate your dining room, and transform your home into an exclusive restaurant experience for one night only.

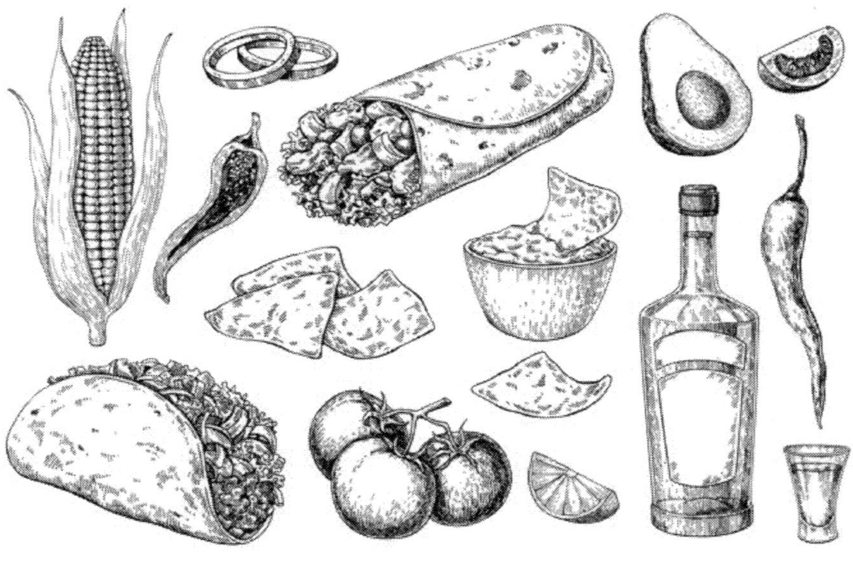

Savoring the Sweet Moments

Retirement doesn't have to be all about sitting at home and watching TV. In fact, it can be a time of adventure and exploration! We explore a variety of activities to add excitement and enjoyment to your retirement years. From trying new hobbies to indulging in guilty pleasures, these ideas are designed to help you create unforgettable memories and make the most of this special time in your life.

- **Sensory deprivation tank -** Experience ultimate relaxation by floating in a sensory deprivation tank. This therapy involves floating in a pod filled with warm salt water, which is designed to block out external stimuli like light and sound.

- **Pole dancing classes -** Get fit while having fun by taking pole dancing classes! Not only is this activity great exercise, but it's also empowering and confidence-building.

- **Nude drawing class -** Embrace your artistic side by taking a nude drawing class. Don't worry if you're not an artist – these classes are designed for beginners and are all about having fun.

- **Tantra workshop -** Explore new levels of intimacy with your partner by attending a tantra workshop. These workshops focus on connecting deeply with your partner through physical touch, breathing exercises, and meditation.

- **Wine tasting class -** Take a wine tasting course to learn about different varietals, regions and pairings. Not only will you expand your knowledge, but you'll get to enjoy some delicious wines as well.

- **Couples massage class -** Learn how to give each other relaxing massages with a couples massage class. This is a great way to bond with your partner while also improving your health and well-being.
- **Burlesque dance classes -** Get in touch with your sensual side by taking burlesque dance classes. These classes are fun, empowering and a great workout.
- **Hot air balloon ride -** Take to the skies in a hot air balloon for an unforgettable experience. You'll get breathtaking views of the landscape below while enjoying a peaceful and serene ride.
- **Tantra retreat -** Go all-in on exploring intimacy and connection by attending a tantra retreat. These multi-day events offer workshops, activities and opportunities to connect deeply with yourself and others.
- **Stand-up comedy class -** Learn how to make people laugh with a stand-up comedy class. This is a great way to boost your confidence, meet new people and have fun.
- **Salsa dance lessons -** Get moving and learn some new moves with salsa dance lessons. This is a great way to stay active, socialize and have fun with your partner or friends.
- **Nude beach visit -** Enjoy the freedom of sunbathing without any tan lines by visiting a nude beach. Just make sure to do your research beforehand and follow proper etiquette!
- **Couples cooking class -** Learn how to cook delicious meals together with a couples cooking class. You'll get to bond

over food and create some tasty dishes that you can enjoy together.

- **Sensual yoga classes -** Connect with your body and explore sensuality through yoga classes designed specifically for this purpose. These classes incorporate movement, breath work, meditation and mindfulness techniques.

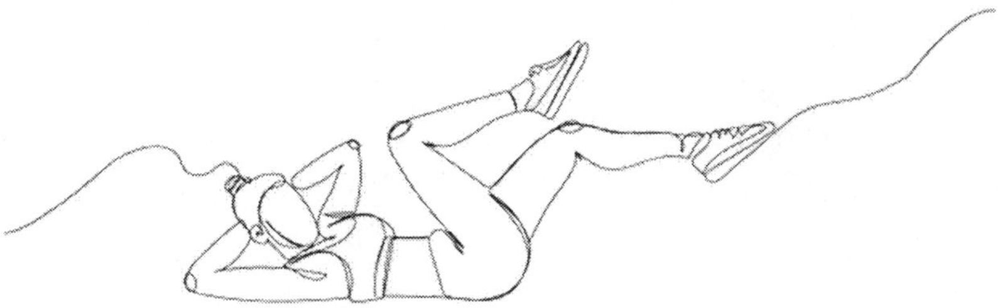

Discover the Joy of Dancing

It's time to embrace all the opportunities that come your way. One such opportunity is dancing! Whether you're a seasoned dancer or a complete beginner, there are plenty of ways to get moving and grooving in retirement. In this chapter, we'll explore some exciting dance activities that will keep you active and engaged in your community. Get ready to put on your dancing shoes and let's hit the dance floor!

- **Swing into the 1920s -** Take a step back in time by learning how to swing dance! Many local dance studios offer classes in this fun and energetic style of dance that originated in the 1920s. You'll be transported back to the era of flappers and speakeasies as you learn how to Lindy Hop, Jitterbug, and Charleston.

- **Line Dancing Marathon -** Get your cowboy boots on and join a line dancing marathon! These events can last anywhere from a few hours to an entire day, with participants dancing non-stop to a variety of country music hits. Not only will you get a great workout, but you'll also meet new people who share your love for this popular form of dance.
- **Ballroom Blitz -** Put on your fanciest attire and attend a ballroom dance competition! Whether you're an experienced dancer or just starting out, these events offer a chance to watch some of the best dancers in the world compete for top honors. And who knows? You may even be inspired to try out some new moves yourself!
- **Belly Dancing Bonanza -** Discover the art of belly dancing with a class or workshop focused on this ancient form of dance. Not only is it great exercise for your core muscles, but it's also a fun way to connect with your inner goddess! Plus, there's something empowering about being able to shimmy and shake like Shakira.
- **Flash Mob Frenzy -** Join a flash mob group and surprise unsuspecting crowds with impromptu dance performances! These groups typically rehearse together before staging surprise performances in public places such as malls or parks. It's a great way to get outside your comfort zone and bring joy and entertainment to others through dance.
- **Cultural Dance Immersion -** Take a trip around the world without leaving your hometown by immersing yourself in different cultural dance styles. Attend a traditional Indian Bharatanatyam class, learn the graceful movements of Chinese fan dancing,

or try out the lively rhythms of African tribal dances.

- **Tap Dancing Troupe -** Join a tap dancing troupe and perform at local events and festivals! Tap dancing is not only fun and entertaining, but it also provides great exercise for your legs and feet. Plus, you'll get to be part of a team that shares your passion for this classic form of dance.

- **Salsa Sensation -** Spice things up by learning how to salsa dance! Salsa classes are available at many community centers and dance studios, and they're a great way to meet new people while getting some exercise. Plus, once you've mastered the basic steps, you can hit up salsa clubs and show off your moves on the dance floor.

- **Musical Theater Madness -** Bring out your inner Broadway star by joining a musical theater group! These groups typically perform classic shows such as "West Side Story" or "Chicago" and require singers who can also dance. Not only will you have fun singing and performing, but you'll also get to work with other talented performers.

- **Square Dancing Soiree -** Put on your best western wear and join a square dancing group! This type of folk dancing is popular all around the country and involves groups of four couples moving together in intricate patterns. It's not only fun but also improves coordination, balance, and cardiovascular health.

- **Dance Fitness Fusion -** Get a full-body workout while having fun with dance fitness fusion classes! These classes combine dance moves with aerobics and strength training exercises for a well-rounded workout. You can find classes in various styles such as Zumba, Cardio Dance, or Hip Hop Fitness.

- **Argentine Tango Adventure -** Experience the passion and elegance of Argentine Tango by taking lessons or attending milongas (tango social dances). This type of tango is known for its close embrace and intricate footwork, making it both challenging and rewarding to learn.
- **Flamenco Fiesta -** Immerse yourself in the fiery rhythms and dramatic movements of flamenco dancing! Take a class or attend a performance to witness the artistry and emotion that goes into this traditional Spanish dance style.
- **Pole Dancing Party** - Challenge yourself physically and mentally by trying out pole dancing! While it may have once been associated with strip clubs, pole dancing has become a popular form of fitness that promotes strength, flexibility, and confidence. Gather some friends for a fun pole dancing party at home or take a class at a studio.
- **Bollywood Blast -** Get ready to move your hips and hands in the colorful world of Bollywood dancing! This energetic dance style originates from Indian films and combines traditional Indian folk dances with modern influences. Take a class or attend an event to experience the joyous music and vibrant costumes that come with Bollywood dancing.

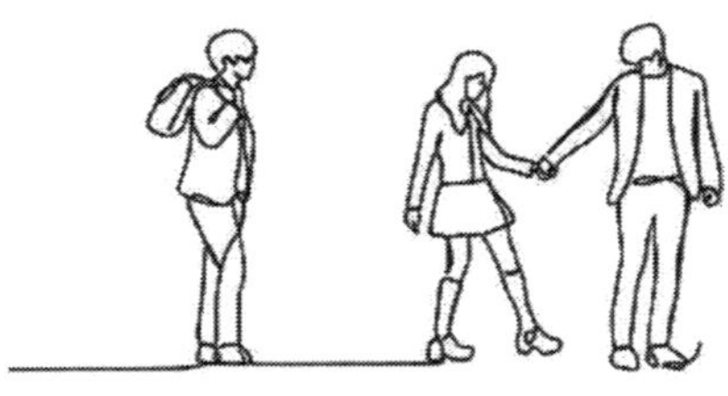

Exploring Festivals, Fairs, and Cultural Events

Experience the vibrant culture of your community through festivals, fairs, and other events! From music festivals to food fairs, these gatherings offer a chance to immerse yourself in local traditions and make new connections. This chapter will guide you through some of the most exciting events to attend during your retirement.

- **Renaissance Fairs -** Step back in time and immerse yourself in the world of knights, jesters, and maidens fair. Renaissance fairs offer a unique opportunity to experience life as it was in the Middle Ages. From jousting competitions to turkey legs, there's something for everyone at these events.

- **Hot Air Balloon Festivals -** Take to the skies and enjoy breathtaking views of the countryside at a hot air balloon festival. These events feature dozens of brightly colored balloons taking off and landing throughout the day. You can even book a ride for an unforgettable experience.

- **Food Truck Rallies -** Sample cuisine from around the world without ever leaving your city at a food truck rally. These events bring together dozens of food trucks serving up everything from tacos to sushi. With live music and entertainment, it's a fun way to spend an afternoon or evening.

- **Oktoberfest Celebrations -** Raise a stein and celebrate German culture at an Oktoberfest event. These festivals feature traditional Bavarian food, music, dancing, and of course beer! Put on your lederhosen or dirndl and join in on the festivities.

- **Lantern Festivals -** Experience the magic of lanterns lighting up the night sky at one of these events. Participants release lanterns into the air with wishes written on them, creating a beautiful display that's sure to leave you feeling inspired.
- **Balloon Glow Events -** Similar to hot air balloon festivals, balloon glow events feature dozens of balloons lighting up the night sky from the ground. It's a magical experience that's sure to leave you in awe.
- **Harvest Festivals -** Celebrate the bounty of fall at a harvest festival. These events typically feature pumpkin patches, corn mazes, hayrides, and apple picking. It's a great way to get outdoors and enjoy the crisp autumn air.
- **Comic Book Conventions -** Embrace your inner geek at a comic book convention. These events bring together fans of all ages to celebrate comics, movies, TV shows, and more. With cosplay contests and celebrity panels, it's a fun way to indulge in your favorite fandoms.
- **Christmas Markets -** Get into the holiday spirit at a Christmas market. These markets feature vendors selling handmade crafts and gifts, as well as delicious food and drink options like mulled wine and gingerbread cookies.
- **Cultural Festivals -** Experience different cultures without leaving your hometown at a cultural festival. From Chinese New Year celebrations to Dia de los Muertos festivities, there are plenty of opportunities to learn about traditions from around the world.

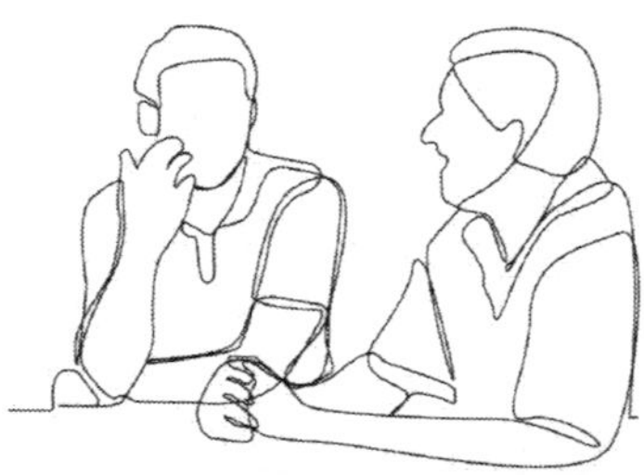

- **Wine and Food Festivals -** Savor the flavors of local cuisine paired with delicious wines at a wine and food festival. These events offer a chance to taste unique dishes prepared by talented chefs while enjoying live music and entertainment.
- **Film Festivals -** Celebrate the art of cinema at a film festival. These events showcase a variety of films from around the world, including independent films and documentaries. With Q&A sessions with filmmakers and actors, it's a great way to deepen your appreciation for movies.
- **State Fairs -** Experience the best of your state at a state fair. From carnival rides to animal exhibits, these fairs offer something for everyone. Indulge in classic fair food like funnel cakes and corn dogs, or try something new like deep-fried Oreos.
- **Art Festivals -** Immerse yourself in creativity at an art festival. These events feature works by local artists in a variety of mediums including painting, sculpture, photography, and more. You can even purchase pieces to add to your own collection.
- **Music Festivals -** Dance the day (or night) away at a music festival. From rock to country to jazz, there are festivals catering to all types of music lovers. Bring a blanket or chair and enjoy performances by your favorite bands or discover new ones.

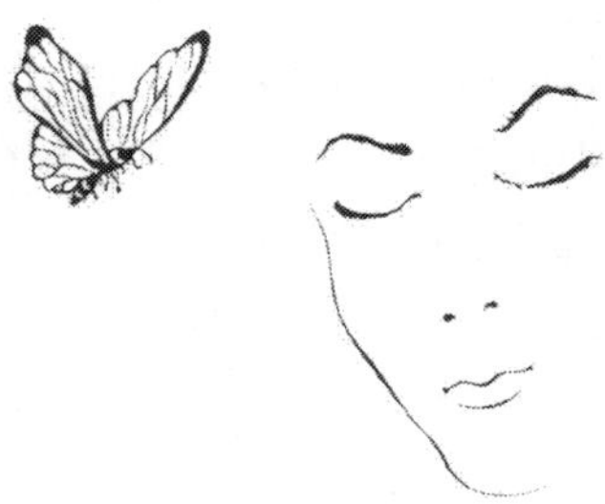

Fun and Fulfilling at the Same Time

Retirement is a time for relaxation, reflection, and enjoying the fruits of your labor. But it's also an opportunity to give back to the world in your own unique way. In this chapter, we'll explore activities that not only bring joy and fulfillment to your life but also make a positive impact on those around you. Get ready to discover the perfect balance between fun and purpose!

- **Voluntourism -** Combine travel with doing good in the world by volunteering abroad. Spend time teaching English to kids in Thailand, building houses in Guatemala or working with animals in Africa.

- **Adopt a Grandparent –** You think you are old now? Not yet. Many elderly people in retirement homes don't have family or friends who visit them regularly. Consider "adopting" a grandparent by visiting with them, bringing them small gifts, or simply spending time with them. It's a great way to make a difference in someone's life while also making new friends.

- **Guerrilla Gardening -** Do you have an empty lot or neglected corner in your neighborhood? Grab some gardening tools and start planting! Guerrilla gardening involves taking over unused public spaces and turning them into beautiful gardens for all to enjoy. Not only will it beautify your community, but it will also help the environment by providing more green space.

- **Volunteer at an Animal Shelter -** If you're an animal lover, consider volunteering at your local animal shelter. You can help care for the animals, walk dogs, or even foster pets until they find their forever homes. Not only will you be helping animals in need, but you'll also get plenty of cuddles and love in return.

- **Storytelling -** Share your life experiences and wisdom with others by becoming a storyteller. You can volunteer at schools, libraries, or retirement homes to share your stories and inspire others.

- **Clean Up Your Local Beach -** If you live near the coast, consider organizing a beach clean-up day with friends and family. Not only will you be helping the environment by removing trash from the beach, but it's also a great way to get some exercise and enjoy the beautiful scenery.

- **Join a Community Garden -** If you enjoy gardening, join a community garden in your area. You'll have access to fresh produce while also getting to know other members of your community.

- **Become an Advocate for a Cause -** Is there a cause that you're passionate about? Consider becoming an advocate or activist for that cause by attending rallies, writing letters to politicians, or even starting your own nonprofit organization.

- **Host A Fundraiser -** Organize a fundraiser for a local charity or nonprofit organization that you support. It could be as simple as hosting a bake sale or as elaborate as planning a gala event. Not only will you be raising money for a good cause, but it's also an opportunity to bring people together and have fun while doing something meaningful.

- **Mentor a Young Person -** Share your knowledge and experience with the next generation by becoming a mentor to a young person in your community. You can volunteer at schools, youth centers, or even start your own mentoring program.

- **Organize A Neighborhood Cleanup -** Get together with your neighbors and organize a cleanup day for your neighborhood. Pick up litter, trim overgrown bushes, and plant flowers to make your community look beautiful.

- **Start A Book Club -** If you love reading, start a book club with friends or join an existing one in your community. It's a great way to stay engaged with literature while also socializing and making new friends.

- **Participate In Citizen Science -** Citizen science projects allow ordinary people to contribute to scientific research by collecting data on topics like bird migration patterns or water quality. Search online for citizen science projects that interest you and get involved!

- **Host A Cultural Exchange -** Invite people from different cultural backgrounds into your home or organize an event where people can share their customs, traditions, and food with each other. It's a great way to learn about other cultures while also building bridges between communities.

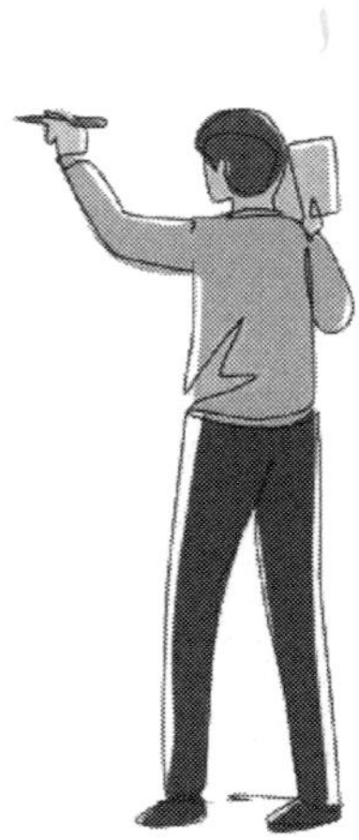

Exciting Activities That Promise a Lot of Thrill

Embrace new experiences that bring excitement and thrill. This chapter explores activities that promise just that, pushing you out of your comfort zone and creating unforgettable memories in the process. From adrenaline-fueled adventures to bucket-list worthy excursions, get ready for a wild ride.

- **Indoor Skydiving -** Experience the rush of skydiving without having to jump out of a plane! Indoor skydiving simulates the feeling of freefall in a vertical wind tunnel, making it safe and accessible for people of all ages. You'll be able to float on air and perform tricks with the help of an instructor.
- **Bungee Jumping -** If you're looking for an adrenaline-pumping activity, bungee jumping might be just the thing for you. Leap off a platform and feel the exhilaration as you plunge towards the ground before being bounced back up by the bungee cord. It's not for the faint-hearted, but it's sure to be an unforgettable experience.
- **Whitewater Rafting -** Get your heart racing with whitewater rafting, where you'll navigate rapids and waves in a raft with a team of fellow adventurers. It's a great way to enjoy nature while also getting an adrenaline fix.
- **Ziplining -** Take in breathtaking views from high above as you soar through the air on a zipline. Whether you're flying over treetops or across canyons, ziplining is sure to give you an unforgettable rush.
- **Hang Gliding -** Soar like a bird and feel the wind rushing

through your hair with hang gliding. You'll be suspended in the air by a lightweight aircraft as you glide over mountains or beaches. It's an experience that will make you feel truly alive.

- **Paragliding -** Similar to hang gliding, paragliding involves flying through the air with a parachute-like wing attached to your body. You can take off from mountains or hillsides and enjoy stunning views as you glide through the sky.
- **Off-Roading -** For those who love adventure on land, off-roading is an exciting way to explore rugged terrain in a 4x4 vehicle or ATV. You'll navigate rough trails and obstacles as you enjoy the thrill of speed and power.
- **Zorbing -** Experience the thrill of rolling down hills inside a giant inflatable ball called a zorb! This unique activity originated in New Zealand but has since spread around the world as an exhilarating way to have fun outdoors.
- **Heli-Skiing -** Take skiing to new heights by being dropped off by helicopter at remote mountain locations for fresh powder runs down steep slopes inaccessible by ski lifts!
- **Kite Surfing –** Combine surfing skills with kite flying skills on this thrilling water sport where strong winds propel riders across waves while they perform tricks in mid-air!
- **Ice Climbing –** Scale frozen waterfalls using ice axes, crampons and ropes! Ice climbing is both physically challenging and mentally stimulating as climbers strategize their ascent up vertical ice walls.

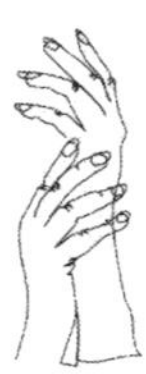

Hilarious Activities You Should Do Once in Your Life

As we grow older, we tend to take life too seriously. We forget that laughter is the best medicine and that sometimes, the most memorable moments are the ones where we let loose and have a good time. In this chapter, we explore some of the funniest activities you can try out in your newfound freedom. From silly pranks to outrageous adventures, get ready to laugh until your sides hurt.

- **Attend a Laughter Yoga Class -** Laughter yoga is a unique activity that combines laughter exercises with deep breathing techniques to promote health and well-being. It's a great way to relieve stress, boost your mood, and have some fun. Find a laughter yoga class in your area and give it a try. You'll be surprised at how good you feel afterwards.

- **Participate in a Flash Mob -** Joining a flash mob is an exciting way to do something spontaneous and silly. Get together with a group of friends or find one online, choose a fun dance routine, and surprise unsuspecting strangers with your moves. Just make sure to practice beforehand so you don't embarrass yourself too much.

- **Attend a Comedy Improv Show -** Watching professional comedians perform improv comedy is always hilarious, but have you ever tried it yourself? Look for local classes or workshops where you can learn the basics of improv comedy and hone your skills in front of an audience.

- **Host a Game Night with Funny Games -** Invite some friends over for a night of board games, but choose ones that are guaranteed to make everyone laugh out loud. Games like Cards Against Humanity, Exploding Kittens, or What Do You

Meme? are perfect for this kind of gathering.

- **Take Part in a Stand-up Comedy Open Mic Night -** If you've always wanted to try stand-up comedy but never had the nerve, retirement is the perfect time to give it a shot. Look for open mic nights at local comedy clubs or bars and sign up for your five minutes of fame on stage. Who knows? You might just discover your hidden talent for making people laugh.

- **Organize a Prank Day -** Gather a group of friends and plan a day of harmless pranks on each other or unsuspecting strangers. Make sure everyone is in on the joke and keep it lighthearted, but don't be afraid to get creative with your pranks.

- **Try Stand-up Paddleboarding Yoga -** Combine two fun activities by trying stand-up paddleboarding yoga. It's a challenging and hilarious way to work on your balance while surrounded by water and nature. Look for classes or guided tours in your area.

- **Attend a Drag Show -** Experience the glitz, glamour, and humor of drag performers at a live show. You'll be entertained by outrageous costumes, sassy lip-syncing, and witty banter that will leave you laughing all night long.

- **Host a Karaoke Party -** Gather some friends, choose your favorite songs, and belt out some tunes at a karaoke party. It's a great way to let loose, have fun, and maybe even discover some hidden musical talent among your group.

- **Join an Improv Everywhere Mission -** Improv Everywhere is a New York City-based prank collective that specializes in staging hilarious public scenes and performances. Check out their website for upcoming events or join their mailing list to be notified about future missions in your area.

- **Take a Comedy Writing Class -** If you have a knack for humor and want to develop your comedy writing skills, consider taking a class or workshop on the subject. You'll learn about joke structure, comedic timing, and how to turn everyday experiences into hilarious stories.
- **Attend a Stand-up Comedy Roast Battle -** Roast battles are events where comedians insult each other in a lighthearted way, often using clever wordplay and witty comebacks. It's a fun and unique way to experience live comedy and see some of the best comedians in action.
- **Go to an Improv Comedy Festival -** Improv comedy festivals bring together performers from all over the world to showcase their talents and compete in various challenges and games. It's a great opportunity to see some of the most creative and hilarious improv acts around.
- **Play Costume Dodgeball -** Take dodgeball to the next level by playing in costume! Choose your favorite character or theme, dress up accordingly, and have fun dodging balls while looking ridiculous.
- **Watch a Puppet Show for Adults -** Puppet shows aren't just for kids anymore! Many puppeteers create shows that are geared towards adults with mature themes, biting satire, and plenty of laughs. Look for shows at local theaters or performing arts venues near you.

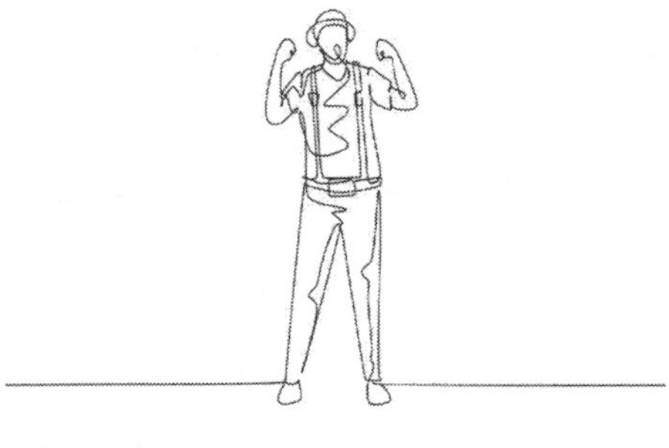

Funny Retirement Prank Ideas to Surprise Your Friends and Family

Retirement is the perfect time to let loose and have some fun, but these activities might not be for the faint of heart. If you're looking for a way to shake things up and push boundaries, we'll explore some unique and disturbingly funny prank ideas that are sure to add a little spice to your newfound freedom. But be warned, these pranks are not for the faint of heart and should not be tested.

- **Clothing Optional Karaoke -** Take karaoke night to another level by stripping down to your birthday suit while belting out your favorite tunes.
- **Fake Your Own Death -** Live out your wildest spy fantasies by faking your own death and observing how people react. Just make sure to come back before too much havoc is wreaked.
- **Host a Seance -** Summon the spirits of the dead and see what kind of mischief they can get up to during an otherworldly game night.
- **Dumpster Diving -** Embrace your inner scavenger by exploring the trash bins in your neighborhood. You never know what treasures you might find!
- **Trespassing Tours -** Explore the forbidden areas of your city by sneaking into abandoned buildings, construction sites, and other off-limits areas.
- **Inappropriate Greeting Cards -** Create a line of greeting cards with inappropriate messages that are sure to shock and offend your loved ones.
- **Prank Call Your Exes -** Get revenge on those who wronged

you in the past by prank calling them with fake accents and outrageous stories.

- **Extreme Couponing -** Take couponing to the next level by hoarding massive amounts of discounted items and turning your home into a veritable warehouse.
- **Staged Public Fights -** Stage public fights with your friends in crowded areas like malls or parks, complete with fake blood and screaming matches.
- **Dumpster Diving Dinners -** Host dinner parties where all the food is sourced from dumpsters around town. You'll be surprised at how delicious discarded food can be!
- **Naked Paintball -** Take your paintball game to the next level by playing in the nude. Just make sure to protect your sensitive areas!
- **Fake Tourist Scams -** Play tourist in your own city and try out different scamming techniques on unsuspecting locals.
- **Extreme Haunted House Visits -** Seek out the scariest haunted houses in your area and see if you can handle their most extreme scares.
- **Public Nudity Pranks -** Stage public nudity pranks in crowded areas like parks or beaches, but don't forget to wear flesh-colored underwear for plausible deniability.
- **Offensive Baking -** Bake offensive treats like anatomically correct gingerbread men or cupcakes with graphic designs for a shockingly sweet twist.

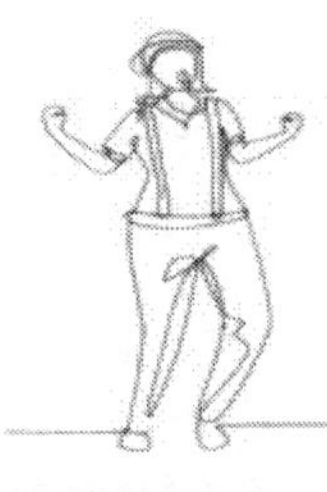

Crazy Ideas That You Should Only Try When Drunk

Don't do it. Seriously.

- **Karaoke Roulette -** Go to a karaoke bar with a group of friends and take turns spinning a wheel with different genres of music. Whatever genre the wheel lands on, you have to choose a song from that category and perform it on stage, no matter how well (or poorly) you know the lyrics. This is sure to lead to some hilarious and unforgettable performances.

- **DIY Slip 'N Slide -** Set up a slip 'n slide in your backyard using plastic sheeting, dish soap, and water. But instead of just sliding down like normal, add some crazy obstacles like inflatable pool toys or giant beach balls to dodge while sliding. Just make sure to have plenty of towels nearby for when you inevitably wipe out.

- **Human Bowling -** Find an empty hallway or long stretch of pavement and set up some empty soda bottles at one end. Then have someone sit in an office chair at the other end while others take turns pushing them towards the bottles like a human bowling ball. Bonus points if you wear ridiculous costumes or use silly sound effects as you roll towards your targets.

- **Blindfolded Taste Test -** Blindfold yourself (or have someone else blindfold you) and try different food items while guessing what they are. You can make it more challenging by using unusual foods or combining flavors that don't typically go together. Just make sure to have some water nearby in case things get too spicy!

- **Painting Party -** Gather some canvases, paint, and brushes and invite some friends over for a painting party after a few drinks. The catch? You have to paint with your non-dominant hand or with your eyes closed for added difficulty (and hilarity). Bonus points if you turn on some music and dance around while painting!
- **Backyard B-Movie Night -** Set up an outdoor movie screen in your backyard and invite friends over for a movie night under the stars. Choose an unconventional movie like a B-movie horror flick or an old-school kung-fu movie that's so bad it's good.

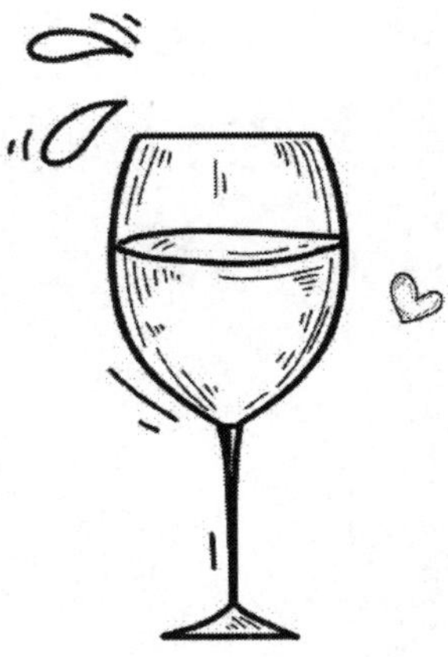

CONCLUSION

Congratulations, you have made it to the end of " Make Your First Year of Retirement Unforgettable". I hope this book has provided you with plenty of inspiration for your retirement journey.

As you begin this new chapter in your life, remember that retirement is not just about relaxing and taking it easy. It's also about pursuing your passions, trying new things, and staying engaged with the world around you.

One of the biggest misconceptions about retirement is that it's a time to slow down and take it easy. While rest and relaxation are certainly important, they shouldn't be the only focus of your retirement years. In fact, studies have shown that retirees who stay engaged with their communities and pursue their interests are happier and healthier than those who don't.

So, as you move forward into retirement, make sure to approach each day with a sense of purpose and enthusiasm. Whether you choose to travel the world, start a new hobby, or simply spend more time with loved ones, make sure that you're doing something that brings you joy and fulfillment.

Another important aspect of retirement is staying connected with others. Retirement can often lead to feelings of isolation or loneliness if we're not careful. Make sure to stay involved in your community through volunteering or joining clubs or organizations that interest you. And don't forget to keep in touch with family and friends - regular phone calls or visits can do wonders for keeping us connected.

Finally, remember that retirement is a gift - one that not everyone gets to experience. So, make the most of it! Take advantage of every opportunity that comes your way and make each day count.

Thank you for reading "Make Your First Year of Retirement Unforgettable". I wish you all the best on your retirement adventure!

DJTS Publishing
info@djts-publishing.com
ISBN Ebook: 978-3-910634-11-4
ISBN Paperback: 978-3-910634-14-5
ISBN Hardcover: 978-3-910634-13-8
Imprint: DJTS Publishing
Images: Licensed by vectorstock, shutterstock DJTS Publishing

Printed in Great Britain
by Amazon

34777992R00073